# Building and Rewarding Your Team

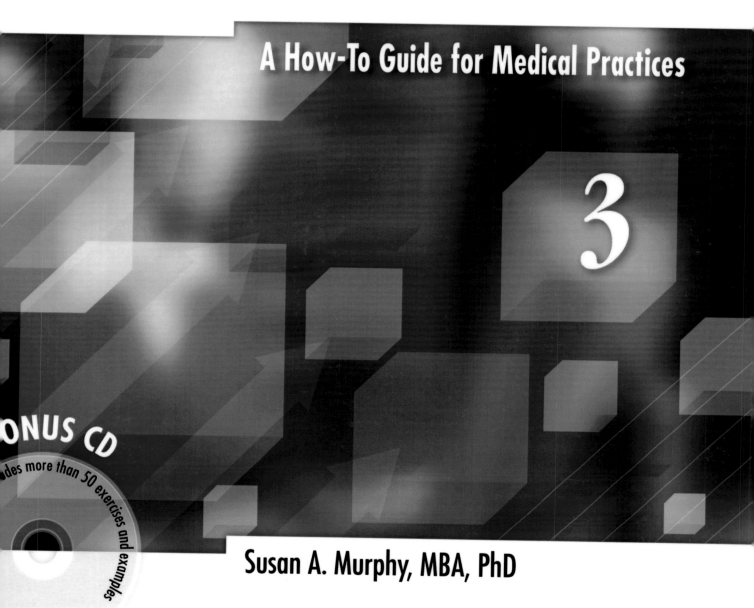

## A How-To Guide for Medical Practices

3

BONUS CD

Includes more than 50 exercises and examples

Susan A. Murphy, MBA, PhD

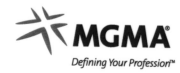

**MGMA®**
*Defining Your Profession™*

Maximizing Performance Management Series

# Building and Rewarding Your Team

## A How-To Guide for Medical Practices

Susan A. Murphy, MBA, PhD

Maximizing Performance Management Series

Medical Group Management Association
104 Inverness Terrace East
Englewood, CO 80112-5306
877.275.6462

mgma.com

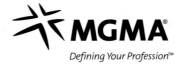

*Production Credits*
Publisher: Marilee E. Aust
Project Editor: Anne Serrano, MA
Copy Editor: Glacier Publishing
Proofreader: Mary Kay Kozyra
Composition: Virginia Howe
Indexer: Sara Lynn Eastler
Cover Design: Jeff Beene

LIBRARY OF CONGRESS CATALOGING-IN-PUBLICATION DATA

Murphy, Susan, 1947-
   Building and rewarding your team : a how-to guide for medical practices / Susan A. Murphy.
      p. ; cm. -- (Maximizing performance management)
   Includes bibliographical references and index.
   Summary: "This book focuses on the connection between performance management and staff engagement in a medical practice. It discusses rewards and recognition and how to evaluate your compensation system. Describing five important performance management components, it offers an appraisal process that directly measures and aligns staff performance with organizational goals"--Provided by publisher.
   ISBN 978-1-56829-327-1
1. Medicine--Practice. 2. Medical personnel. 3. Personnel management. 4. Health care teams. 5. Employee motivation. I. Medical Group Management Association. II. Title. III. Series.
   [DNLM: 1. Employee Incentive Plans. 2. Practice Management, Medical--organization & administration. 3. Group Processes. 4. Reward. W 80 M978b 2009]
   R728.M87 2009
   610.68--dc22
                                   2008033007

Item # 7093

ISBN: 978-1-56829-327-1

Copyright © 2009 Medical Group Management Association

Printed in the United States of America
10 9 8 7 6 5 4 3 2 1

# Acknowledgments

The books in the Maximizing Performance Management Series may have my name on the covers, but they would not exist without the knowledge, enthusiasm, and expertise of many people. Space does not allow me to list everyone, but I want to publicly acknowledge a few colleagues who played especially important roles in the creation of the book you are holding in your hands. Acknowledgments always say "I could not have written this book without their help," but in this case it is absolutely true.

Incentives and compensation are critical components in motivating and rewarding the team, and I turned to two leading experts for help. Laura Jacobs and Mary Witt from the Camden Group contributed this important section. Special thanks go to Steve Valentine, President of the Camden Group, for his enthusiastic support and endorsement of Laura and Mary's participation.

A number of current and former Medical Group Management Association colleagues had special roles in making this series a reality. Marilee Aust understood the importance of this topic during our initial conversation two years ago. Marilee and Anne Serrano, MA are amazing, and the series benefited greatly from their ideas, enthusiasm, and publication skills. I'd also like to thank Julie Sommer, MGMA's talented marketing manager. Drew Di Giovanni and Peg McHugh, formerly with the MGMA, also made important contributions.

Other experts deserve acknowledgment as well for their contributions to different sections of the series. They include: generational guru Claire Raines (the section on generational differences); human resources expert David Milovich (content throughout the series); Matt Mulherin, (success stories as well as the most up-to-date Press Ganey, Inc. research statistics); and Lisa Goddard (editing skills). Real-world case studies make these concepts come alive, and I thank all of those involved including Colleen Conway-Welch, RN, PhD; Deborah W. Royer, MGA; Gene Spiritus, MD; Christy Sandborg, MD; and Bill Zangwill, PhD. Dr. Pat Heim, my mentor and friend for 25 years, generously gave me permission to use information that we developed for our book *In the Company of Women*. Our co-author, Susan Golant, challenges me by example to constantly improve my writing skills.

On the personal front, my husband Jim kept me sane and focused and laughing over the last two years, which was no easy feat. He was my one-man Management Team helping me to maximize my *own* performance while I was writing. I am also blessed with another wonderful support team — my parents, Alice and Bill Applegarth, and my siblings Anne, Ginger, and Paul.

Finally, I am grateful to the thousands of colleagues, clients, friends, and associates with whom I have worked over the years. They have been my best teachers, and I am grateful to now share their real-world lessons with the reader.

# Contents

# CD (TOOLS, HELPING MECHANISMS, AND CASE STUDIES)*

## Tools/Helping Mechanisms

Americans with Disability Act

Anger

Assess Your Outlook

Benchmarking Your Effectiveness

Checking Your Delegating Skills

Compensation System Self-Assessment Tool: 12 Questions for Better Results

Culture Check Procedure

Decisions by Consensus

Disciplinary Action Steps

Equal Employment Opportunity Laws

Example of Cascading Goals

Exercise: Cash on the Spot

Exercise: External Environment

Exercise: How Are You Communicating the Practice's Mission, Values, and Goals?

Exercise: Name that Mission!

Exercise: Practice Dealing With Minor Errors

Exercise: Purposes Critique

Exercise: The Goal Journey

Exercise: Types of Feedback

Exercise: What Else is Going On?

Exercise: Who Else Needs to Know?

Federal Laws and State and Local Laws

Financial Measures—Which to Use?

Goal Planning Tool

Hiring Employees Checklist

How Good Are You at Performance Management?

How to Give Praise

Integrated Performance Self-Assessment Tool

Key Actions to Align Your Developing Team Members with Goals

New Physician Orientation Checklist

Performance Appraisal Checklist for Managers

Performance Counseling Memo for Discipline

Performance/Feasibility Grid

Questions to be Avoided

Quiz: How Well Does Your Organization Manage Change?

Review Resume in Light of Qualifications Necessary

Sample Balance Sheet Outline

Sample Business Plan Outline

Sample Coaching Plan

Sample Code of Conduct

Sample Code of Conduct for Meetings and Interactions

Sample Conflict/Complaint Resolution Policy (includes Conflict/Complaint Resolution Form)

Sample Conflict Resolution Guidelines

Sample Customer Service Quality Standards

Sample Disciplinary Policies and Procedures

Sample Financial Plan Outline

Sample Medical Practice Satisfaction Survey

Sample Meeting Agenda

Sample Meeting Format Critique

Sample Policy on Workplace Harassment

Sample Strategic Plan Outline

Sample Telephone Standards

Sample Values and Norms

Steps for Terminating a Team Member

What Change Is Occurring?

What Is Your Personal Distress Level?

## Case Studies

The Emory Clinic, Inc., Atlanta, Georgia

Emory Healthcare Primary Care Practice in Smyrna, Georgia

Floyd Primary Care, Rome, Georgia

John Muir Medical Center, Walnut Creek, California

Kaiser Permanente, Northern California Strategy

Kaiser Permanente, Northern California Performance Award Program

Press Ganey Best Practices for Medical Groups

Providence Health & Services — Southern California

Saint Mary's Nell J. Redfield Health Centers, Reno, Nevada

University of California — Irvine Medical Center

Vanderbilt University Medical Center and Medical Group

---

* CD includes CD-only material as well as tools and helping mechanisms from all four books in the *Maximizing Performance Management Series.*

# Introduction

As Michael optimistically walks into the Green Valley Medical Group building to report for his first day on the job, he can't help but feel excited. "I've worked so hard to get to this point in my career. I know that I can make a difference in this practice. After all, it used to have the reputation as the best in the city."

It's true that during the interview process, the seven physicians had described a very bleak view of their practice. However, Michael is sure that they were painting an overly negative picture because the last manager had glossed over so many of the problems with patient satisfaction and the staff morale issues, and then to add insult to injury, absconded with $500,000 in cash. Now with the practice on the verge of bankruptcy, the physicians wanted to find a strong manager who would permit them to return to taking care of patients. And Michael knows that he's the right choice. It couldn't be as bad as they represented it. Besides, he's ready for the challenge and has already paid his dues running much smaller practices for the past 15 years.

As Michael steps off the elevator onto the second floor and begins the trek to his new office, he imagines what it's like to be a patient here. Five patients are in the waiting area already, coffee-stained magazines are scattered throughout the room, and two of the patients are talking loudly on cell phones. Michael says "good morning" to the patients as he passes through the private entrance to his new office. Suddenly, Michael is hit by what seems to be a curtain of tension. Karen, the receptionist, has her nose to the computer and grunts at Michael as he greets her with a cheerful "good morning!" Two of the nurses, Ron and Jenna, can't seem to muster any more excitement for Michael's first day either — the two of them appear to be embroiled in their own brawl. "Maybe the physicians weren't exaggerating during my interviews," Michael thought.

"I'll make the rounds and check on the physicians to see how they're doing on my first day here," thought Michael. "They'll probably give me some ideas about where they want me to start." Michael starts with Dr. Samuels, one of the founders of the practice some 20 years ago. As Michael enters her office, he finds her buried under what looks like an explosion of charts, paperwork, personnel files, prescription pads, journal articles, and a plethora of things he can't even decipher. He's reminded of those pictures he's seen on the news of some third-world country after a major disaster has hit — people marshalling any small bit of strength in order to just make it through another day.

After Michael snaps back to the reality that is Dr. Samuels' office, and not a small village after a 9.0 earthquake, his fanciful ideas of riding into a practice on a white horse and cleaning up a few surface-level problems and then basking in the awe of all of his coworkers dies quickly. Michael realizes that he is walking into a workplace that is in need of a major overhaul and that to turn this practice around might be more difficult than building a new practice from scratch. This is no longer a "kick a couple of tires and change the oil" proposition, he has been hired to rebuild the car — but the catch is, he doesn't have the option of buying all of the new parts and just putting it together. He has to decide which parts need the most attention first, take care of them, and then carefully rebuild this machine into a smooth-running, service-oriented, quality organization. And he doesn't have much time.

Throughout the morning, Michael stops by each physician's office, and most of them resemble Dr. Samuels'. As Michael talks to the physicians about their major concerns, many of his first impressions are confirmed by what they say: The office staff is disjointed and unwilling to work with each other. Ron and Jenna just can't seem to get over the different ways in which they communicate — leaving them to pass one another without as much as a glance — and the rest of the staff seems to have joined sides with either Ron or Jenna. More hiring needs to be done, but the physician partners are nervous about hiring any new employees and placing them into this toxic environment. More unhappy employees would make the culture even worse. Patient satisfaction is so low that they have stopped measuring it.

Where should Michael start? It seems like every system in this medical group practice is broken. There is high staff turnover; low morale, low productivity, and low quality; dissatisfied patients; bewildered physicians; and significant financial trouble. Michael decides to begin his journey by taking a systemwide approach that will align team member performance with medical practice goals. By using a systems thinking approach, Michael decides to assess the medical group as a large system with six subsystems that need to be in balance, congruent, and support the medical group's goals.

The subsystems Michael evaluates are from the Weisbord 6 Box model that is discussed in chapter 1. These subsystems include:

- ➤ Purposes (Vision/Mission/Values/Norms/Goals);
- ➤ Leadership;
- ➤ Rewards (and Recognition);
- ➤ Structure;
- ➤ Relationships; and
- ➤ Helping mechanisms.

Each of these subsystems communicates to each team member what is important and how to behave — each subsystem directly impacts patient care. The first step is to define the purposes — the mission, values, and goals — of the medical group. Then Michael must determine which subsystems are not supporting them. Any deficiencies in these subsystems would then be addressed.

On that first day, Michael orders in pizza for the physicians for their lunch break. As he looks at the perplexed faces of his new team of physicians around the conference table, Michael takes a deep breath and officially begins his new job as medical group manager.

Michael begins, "Let's get to work and create a new and improved medical practice. One where you want to practice medicine, your staff wants to work, and your patients want to come for care. Let me start by asking you what you would like your organization to resemble."

"Well," Dr. Black speaks hesitantly, "I just want it to run smoothly."

"But *how exactly* would you like that to look? What are your goals for this practice?" prompts Michael.

"I'll be honest with you," confesses Dr. Samuel, "I don't think I've given it that much thought lately. Isn't that why we hired you?"

"I think it's important that we examine the problems that are affecting your practice currently," reasons Michael. "I know that you physicians are incredibly busy — that's one of the reasons you hired me, but at the end of the day, your names are on that office door. You need to be sure that your staff is a reflection of the type of practice you want to convey to your patients. Rather than mulling over how things haven't gone right, let's focus on the things that are going well in addition to those that need to be rectified so that you can be proud of the practice you've worked so hard to achieve."

Dr. Jordan exclaims, "We agree, Michael. Where do we start?"

Michael explains, "You need to start thinking about what you want your practice to reveal. We're going to rid this practice of its toxicity, and we're going to transform the culture into one that is focused, goal oriented, and people oriented."

Michael spent the next week observing the practice and interviewing every physician and team member about the mission, values, goals, leadership, rewards, structure, relationships, policies, and procedures. After the system assessment, Michael held a strategic planning session for the physicians, senior managers, and stakeholders. After the plan was developed, Michael set out to communicate the objectives to the rest of the staff. The next steps were to align the subsystems with the new goals of the practice.

## LEADERSHIP ROLE IN EMPLOYEE ENGAGEMENT AND RETENTION

Michael voraciously researched the recent studies about employee engagement and retention. He was alarmed to read that the Gallup Poll in 2006 found that only 33 percent of the U.S. workforce is actively engaged, while 15 percent of the workforce is actively disengaged at productivity and quality costs of $328 billion per year![1] When leaders were actively engaged, there was a 14 percent higher engagement of employees and 19 percent higher employee retention — highly engaged employees are much less likely to leave organizations within the next year. Additionally, the poll found that engaged employees are likely to be an organization's best source of new ideas. Michael eagerly shared this information with the physician leadership, insisting that they play an active role in engaging and retaining staff.

Michael continued his research and was surprised by the findings from the Center for Creative Leadership® (CCL) about employee engagement and retention. The CCL found that all generations want similar cultures in their workplace:

- People want recognition and to feel valued;
- Development is the most valued form of recognition, even more so than pay raises and enhanced titles;
- Constant learning on and through the job is what people demand; and
- Almost everyone wants a coach or mentor, and most want their leaders to serve in this role.

Michael pleaded with the physician leaders to fill these needs for the physicians and team members.[2]

During Michael's meetings with the physician leadership, he cited important research by Press Ganey Associates about the top six priorities for health care employees:

- Senior leadership who really listens to employees;
- Enough staff to provide quality care;
- Promotions to be handled fairly;
- Senior leadership who respond promptly to most problems;
- Senior leadership who can be trusted to be straightforward and honest; and
- Involvement in decision making.

Michael found that attracting and retaining younger physicians was one of the key areas of concern for the more-senior members of the medical staff. Michael provided the physicians with the Cejka Search 2006 Physician Retention Survey that reveals factors such as cultural fit and family as driving forces in physician turnover:

➤ "Poor cultural fit" is the single most frequently mentioned reason for physicians to voluntarily leave a practice (51 percent);

➤ Family is a strong contributor to a physician's decision to leave a practice. Reasons that required the physician to relocate were "to be closer to own or spouse's family" (42 percent); and

➤ The need for flexible schedules, less on-call time, and seeking higher compensation were revealed as factors for physicians leaving practices.

Michael emphasized the critical importance of developing a values-driven, relationship-oriented coaching culture where younger physicians receive mentoring support as they begin their medical careers.

## PATIENT SATISFACTION PRIORITIES

Michael has always measured patient satisfaction with the Press Ganey surveys and explained the most recent indices of patient satisfaction to his new medical group. The top six patient priorities include:

➤ Our sensitivity to their needs;

➤ Overall cheerfulness of our practice;

➤ Overall rating of care received during their visit;

➤ Comfort and pleasantness of the exam room;

➤ Waiting time in exam room before being seen by care provider; and

➤ Amount of time the care provider spent with them.

## ALIGNING EMPLOYEE PERFORMANCE WITH ORGANIZATIONAL GOALS

Although this book and the Maximizing Performance Management Series as a whole serve as detailed manuals for building a medical group practice for individuals like Michael, *every* organization has systems that can be improved. (Exhibit I-1 shows the flow from individual team member goals to vision, mission, and values, and back again.) So, even though your practice may not be suffering from poor patient satisfaction or enormous staff morale issues or on the brink of bankruptcy, the system-by-system diagnosis and prescriptions in this book and the series will improve the performance of your practice.

The six subsystems as shown in Exhibit I-2 must be in balance in order to align team member performance with goals. Description and exploration of these subsystems appear in the following books in the Maximizing Performance Management Series:

➤ **Box 1: Purposes:** *Aligning the Team with Practice Goals: A How-To Guide for Medical Practices* (Book 1)

➤ **Box 2: Leadership:** *Leading, Coaching, and Mentoring the Team: A How-To Guide for Medical Practices* (Book 2)

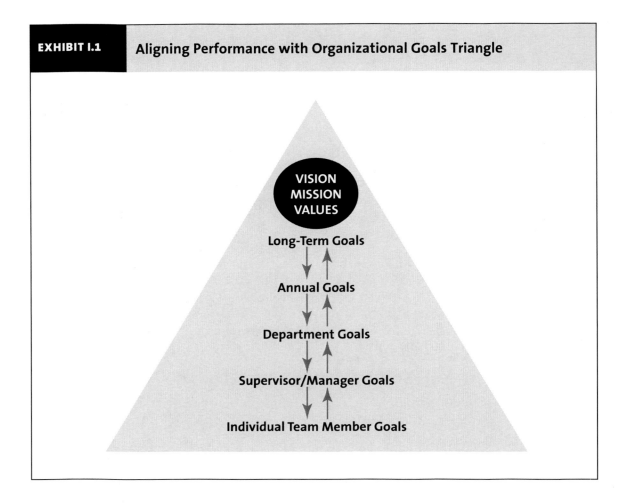

**EXHIBIT I.1**    **Aligning Performance with Organizational Goals Triangle**

VISION
MISSION
VALUES

Long-Term Goals

Annual Goals

Department Goals

Supervisor/Manager Goals

Individual Team Member Goals

> ➤ **Box 3: Rewards and Box 4: Structures:** *Building and Rewarding Your Team: A How-To Guide for Medical Practices* (Book 3)
>
> ➤ **Box 5: Relationships:** *Relationship Management and the New Workforce: A How-To Guide for Medical Practices* (Book 4)
>
> ➤ **Box 6: Resources/Helping Mechanisms: (CD)** (With all books)

Chapter 1, which is the same in each book in the series, explains the systems approach to aligning team member performance with organizational goals. Every medical practice is a dynamic system with six subsystems. For alignment to occur, each of six subsystems must be in balance and consistently support the medical practice goals. If one or more of these subsystems is weak and is not supporting the medical practice goals, the performance of team members cannot be effectively aligned with the goals. In chapter 1, the six subsystems are explained, and diagnostic exercises clearly define areas of strength and weakness.

A brief synopsis of boxes 1 through 6, including chapter contents of each book in the series, follows.

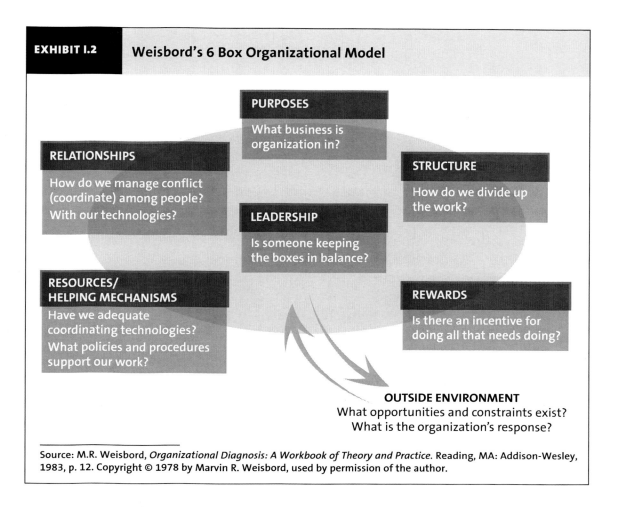

**EXHIBIT I.2** **Weisbord's 6 Box Organizational Model**

**PURPOSES**

What business is organization in?

**RELATIONSHIPS**

How do we manage conflict (coordinate) among people? With our technologies?

**STRUCTURE**

How do we divide up the work?

**LEADERSHIP**

Is someone keeping the boxes in balance?

**RESOURCES/ HELPING MECHANISMS**

Have we adequate coordinating technologies? What policies and procedures support our work?

**REWARDS**

Is there an incentive for doing all that needs doing?

**OUTSIDE ENVIRONMENT**
What opportunities and constraints exist?
What is the organization's response?

Source: M.R. Weisbord, *Organizational Diagnosis: A Workbook of Theory and Practice.* Reading, MA: Addison-Wesley, 1983, p. 12. Copyright © 1978 by Marvin R. Weisbord, used by permission of the author.

## BOX 1: Purposes

*Aligning the Team with Practice Goals: A How-To Guide for Medical Practices* (Book 1)

Chapter 2 explains how to develop the vision, mission, values, norms, and short- and long-term goals for your practice. Chapter 3 explains how to accomplish strategic planning, including the new model of Appreciative Inquiry. Chapter 4 demonstrates how to set SMART goals (specific, measurable, achievable, results-oriented, and time-bound) for each department and how to strategically link each goal to the overall medical practice goals. Next, managers are shown how to cascade the goals developed from the mission throughout the organization and into the individual team member performance plans.

## Box 2: Leadership

*Leading, Coaching, and Mentoring the Team: A How-To Guide for Medical Practices* (Book 2)

The medical practice leadership is crucial for keeping the other subsystems balanced. This section focuses on the roles of the leaders in aligning employee performance with organizational goals. These chapters explore how leaders can effectively "walk the talk" every day and offer several methods for communicating the strategic plan and organizational goals to team members.

Chapter 2 describes the four leadership characteristics that are critical for successful leaders today and the role of emotional intelligence for leaders. Chapter 3 examines the leader's role during change and the fact that although change is inevitable, growth is optional. The four stages for change are described in addition to the leadership actions needed at each stage so that team members can continue to be goal focused despite major changes.

Chapter 4 introduces the Situational Leadership® Model that is a four-stage process for orienting, training, and leading team members by focusing on how well they are aligning their performance with the organization's goals. The four stages are directing, coaching, supporting, and delegating. Through this process, the team member goes from being dependent on the leader for direction in Stage 1 to being more independent in Stage 4, where the leader can both successfully delegate tasks and be assured that the organization goals and objectives are being met. This model ensures that team members know, from their manager, what their goals are and what is expected of them, and then the manager supports the team members as they advance through the development stages in their jobs, culminating in the delegation stage.

Chapter 5 introduces managers to an innovative process whereby a manager can effectively communicate with a team member about his or her inappropriate, non-goal-oriented behavior in a manner that emphasizes both the goals and the performance the manager wants from the team member, and yet does not cause team member defensiveness. This innovative system will effectively address more than 95 percent of team members' inappropriate behaviors and get the team back on track toward goals — it effectively focuses on goals instead of mistakes. Additionally, this innovative system provides a consistent way for managers to discipline team members who are unable or unwilling to align their performance with organizational goals.

Chapter 6 explains how to create a coaching culture where leaders coach the individual team members using a multistep coaching model that includes setting/communicating SMART goals, training team members, building relationships, motivating and using positive reinforcement, monitoring performance, and giving feedback. The goal of the coaching system is to keep both managers and the team focused on aligning performance with organizational goals.

Chapter 7 illustrates how leaders establish a mentoring process for the team, focusing particularly on physician mentoring in both the clinical and academic settings. Young physicians want mentoring and will choose organizations that offer mentoring in order to enhance their skills in the most expeditious way.

# BOX 3: Rewards and BOX 4: Structure

*Building and Rewarding Your Team: A How-To Guide for Medical Practices* (Book 3)

Chapter 2 describes the importance of the rewards and recognition subsystem. It explains the role of compensation and incentives in engaging the team. This important chapter examines what physicians want, how to design an effective compensation system, and how to evaluate your current compensation system's effectiveness.

Chapters 3–6 demonstrate the importance of the structure subsystem. Chapter 3 includes how to interview, select, and hire the most appropriate candidate for the job to be performed. This includes Jim Collins' ideas of getting the right people on the bus and in the right seats. Chapter 4 examines the importance of an excellent team member orientation process, including physician orientation. More than 25 percent of new employees leave within the initial three months; therefore, creating a sound orientation process is critical in aligning employee performance with organizational goals.

Chapter 5 explains the five important components for performance management and how to ensure that each team member's performance aligns with organizational goals. The significant connection between performance management and employee engagement is clarified.

Chapter 6 describes a performance appraisal process that directly measures and aligns team member performance with organizational goals. This chapter discusses the importance of preparation for the performance appraisal meeting through the evaluation to determine the effectiveness of the meeting.

# BOX 5: Relationships

*Relationship Management and the New Workforce: A How-To Guide for Medical Practices* (Book 4)

This book covers the critical subsystem of relationships among the team. Chapters 2, 3, and 4 examine the role of effective conflict management in the medical group practice.

Chapter 2 defines conflict and the cost when it is not managed effectively. Ways to decrease defensiveness are explained and effective conflict management guidelines are proffered to decrease the destructive nature of conflict. Chapter 3 introduces difficult conversation techniques, the difference between content and relationship conflict, as well as the five styles for managing conflict: collaborating, competing, compromising, accommodating, and avoiding.

Chapter 4 includes the role of effective conflict management in team development. The second stage of the team development process, storming, must include healthy conflict or the team development process could be thwarted. Groupthink is discussed, in addition to several types of difficult people who can interfere with aligning team performance with organizational goals.

Chapter 5 introduces gender differences and the importance in organizations of understanding the physiological, genetic, and sociological differences between men and women. These differences are often invisible to us and can cause conflict in organizations because men and women often have differences in how they communicate, make decisions, manage meetings, and view the world.

Chapter 6 introduces generational differences and explains how the four generations in the workplace today have been raised on different planets in many respects. The World War II generation, Baby Boomers, Generation Xers, and Millennials have different viewpoints about leadership, work ethic, teamwork, technology, and many other areas. By understanding the different viewpoints of these generations, leaders can be more effective in maximizing team performance. Chapter 6 reveals the actions that practices can take to attract and retain physicians and other team members of all generations.

## BOX 6:  Resources/Helping Mechanisms *(CD)*

These files contain many resources and tools, including procedures for managing conflict, guidelines for customer service quality standards, policies for employee discipline, and employment process checklists. Also included are several case studies that demonstrate excellence in efforts to align team performance with organizational goals.

Press Ganey Award winners include practices that have decreased patient waiting time, increased patient education about radiation and chemotherapy, improved patient billing, and enhanced team member satisfaction and sense of ownership.

Vanderbilt University Medical Group, University of California-Irvine Medical Center, and Kaiser Permanente Medical Group in Northern California are highlighted in depth to demonstrate their successful efforts to align team performance with organizational goals.

The bottom line is that this comprehensive, results-oriented book provides a road map and prescriptions to take you and your medical practice to the next level and beyond. Whether you want to fine-tune your practice or manage a complete overhaul of the entire operation, this book provides the answers you need to align the performance of your team with your practice goals.

# REFERENCES

[1] The Gallup Organization, "Employee Engagement Index," *The Gallup Management Journal* (October 2006).

[2] R. Plettnix, *Emerging Leader: Implications for Engagement and Retention.* (Brussels, Belgium: Center for Creative Leadership, 2006).

## CHAPTER 1

# Systems Approach · · · · · · · · · · · · · · · · · · · · · · · · · · · · · · · · · · · · · · · · · · · · · ·

Organizations are like humans. Both organizations and humans are systems made up of many subsystems — and each of these subsystems contributes to the overall health of the entity.

What exactly is a system? A system is a collection of things that interact with each other to function as a whole. There are many types of systems: biological, ecological, families, cities, the universe, businesses, governments, hospitals, and medical practices, to name a few.

Experts in health care are now taking a more holistic approach when assessing the health of a person by looking at all the systems in the body. And experts in organizations now look at all the systems in the organization to assess its overall health. This approach is known as systems thinking. Systems thinking is a holistic approach to viewing an organization, to understand how all parts of a system are linked together.

In our human bodies, each organ, bone, muscle, and nerve plays a unique part within the whole body. A strong contribution from one component can't make up for deficiencies in the others.

It's impossible to diagnose the overall health of a person by examining merely one component. Body functions are integrated and their interactions are as important as their individual roles. General practitioner physicians have become the gatekeepers in many medical practices, so all the systems of the whole body can be viewed in a more holistic manner. Specialists are often brought in later to treat individual components that are diseased.

This systems approach to the body can be applied to assessing the health of organizations. The model I like to use in my holistic diagnosis of organizations was developed by Marvin Weisbord and it's called the 6 Box Organizational Model (see Exhibit 1.1). It provides a holistic view of an organization. I think of it as viewing the total system, and its subsystems, from an altitude of 35,000 feet.

The six "boxes" are:

1. Purposes;

2. Leadership;

3. Rewards;

4. Structure;

5. Relationships; and

6. Resources/Helping Mechanisms.

As seen in the diagram, there's a seventh component that complicates these six internal interactions. That seventh component is the external environment. An organization is an "open system," and it cannot be static. As we'll discuss in more detail later, leaders of organizations must be aware of what's occurring externally, that is, outside of their organizations, and these leaders must be proactive. Jack Welch, former chief executive officer (CEO) of General Electric, said, "If the amount of change inside an organization is less than the amount of change outside, then the end is in sight." The rate of change is accelerating and continuously impacts what is occurring inside organizations.

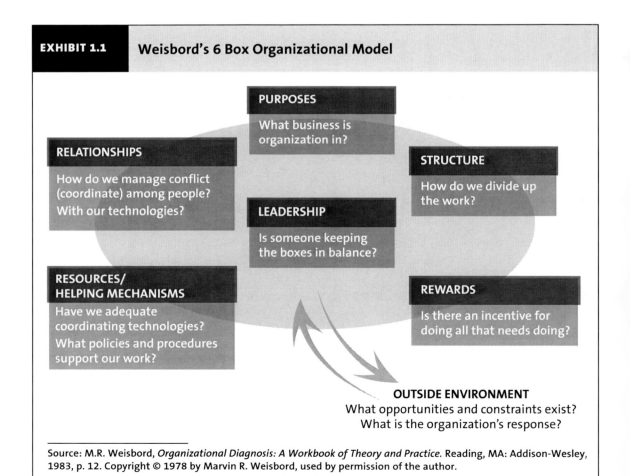

**EXHIBIT 1.1    Weisbord's 6 Box Organizational Model**

**PURPOSES**
What business is organization in?

**RELATIONSHIPS**
How do we manage conflict (coordinate) among people? With our technologies?

**STRUCTURE**
How do we divide up the work?

**LEADERSHIP**
Is someone keeping the boxes in balance?

**RESOURCES/ HELPING MECHANISMS**
Have we adequate coordinating technologies? What policies and procedures support our work?

**REWARDS**
Is there an incentive for doing all that needs doing?

**OUTSIDE ENVIRONMENT**
What opportunities and constraints exist?
What is the organization's response?

Source: M.R. Weisbord, *Organizational Diagnosis: A Workbook of Theory and Practice.* Reading, MA: Addison-Wesley, 1983, p. 12. Copyright © 1978 by Marvin R. Weisbord, used by permission of the author.

# THIS MODEL WORKS

I've been using the Weisbord 6 Box model to align organizational goals and behavior for 25 years. During the 1980s, I used this model as the organization diagnostic tool for 20 health care facilities when I worked at American Medical International, Inc. (AMI), as an internal consultant. This model can be used in any type of organization. In fact, in my current consulting practice, I've used this model successfully in many industries, including medical and legal practices, hospitals, manufacturing, technology, public relations, research, government, and academia.

In conducting my diagnosis, I analyze the organization using each of the six boxes. I interview managers and team members, asking them questions about the mission and values, leadership, rewards and recognition, structure, relationships, and helping mechanisms throughout the organization.

Several years ago I was part of a "dream team" whose project was to work in a think tank and build the "hospital of the future." This dream team consisted of six individuals — the CEO, four vice presidents, and an organization development consultant (me). Although I started as a consultant on this project, I was fortunate to join the team as a vice president when the medical center opened. We had the prodigious opportunity to build both the physical plant and the organization systems from the beginning. During the two years it took to build the physical structure, we meticulously created the organization building blocks one by one.

We started from scratch — all we had was a big chunk of land in Orange County, California. AMI was bankrolling this project.

We dreamed that our hospital of the future was to be a value-based organization that included systems designed so that everything about the organization — the people, the building lay-out, the medical staff, the volunteers — was aligned to meet our organizational goals. We created an organization based on values and then created systems so that those values were reinforced and communicated throughout every part of the organization, including goal setting, physician recruitment, patient satisfaction, conflict management practices, as well as hiring, rewarding, coaching, promoting, and firing employees.

We used this 6 Box organizational model as the framework for building our hospital of the future. Within the first year of operation, there was immediate quantifiable success. For example, our medical center received several top awards from the corporate office when measured against the other 125 health care centers throughout the United States:

- #1 in patient satisfaction;
- #1 in physician satisfaction; and
- #1 in employee satisfaction.

There were other signs of success: *Modern Healthcare* magazine named our CEO, John Gaffney, Administrator of the Year. The facility received a full three-year accreditation from the Joint Commission for Accreditation of Health Organizations (JCAHO) during the initial year opening. We had been hoping for one year! JCAHO referred other hospitals to us for help. McGraw-Hill published a book about our hospital of the future: *The Orders of Change: Building Value-Driven Organizations,* written by R.L. Kennedy © 1995.

## OVERVIEW OF THE 6 BOX MODEL

Let's examine each of these six boxes, or subsystems, in a generic way by demonstrating the kinds of questions that need consistent answers in order to align team performance with organizational goals. Later in this chapter, I'll elaborate and provide more examples about how to utilize these subsystems in medical practices.

### Purposes (Vision/Mission/Values/Norms/Goals)

What "business" are we in? What are we attempting to accomplish? What values should guide our operating processes and are critical to our culture and our success? How are we going to treat each other and our patients?

What are our short-term and long-term goals? Are the purpose, mission, values, and goals aligned so that they are clear and do not contradict one another?

### Leadership

Is someone keeping the other boxes in balance? Who is connecting the vision, mission, and values to the strategy, structure, and systems? Who is developing our culture and empowering, enabling, and energizing the team? Who is communicating the purpose, mission, values, and goals? Are all the leaders communicating similar messages through their actions and words? What happens when one of the leaders does not demonstrate that s/he agrees with the purpose, mission, values, and goals? Is there continual coaching and continuous improvement toward the goals?

### Rewards

Is there an incentive for doing all that needs to be done? What's in it for the staff to support our purpose? Are we measuring the outcomes that tie directly to our mission and goals? Are we rewarding the values and behaviors that we want? For example, if we say that teamwork is one of our values, are we rewarding only individual accomplishments?

## Structure

How do we divide the work? Is staffing adequate? Do we have enough staff members to provide quality work? How many sites do we need in order to achieve our purpose? Are people trained to do the work they are assigned to do so that we can achieve our mission and values? Are the roles and responsibilities clear? Is the workflow design efficient and effective with the most appropriate people performing the job assignments? Does the organizational design prevent duplication of efforts as well as stop assignments from falling through the cracks?

## Relationships

How do we manage conflict among people? How do we manage conflict with our technologies? What are relationships like? Is communication open, authentic, and plentiful to align everyone toward the goals? Is teamwork encouraged at all levels? Does the culture of the organization foster trust and collaboration? How are conflicts dealt with among the constituents? For example, in health care, what happens when there are disagreements and conflict among physicians, staff, patients, or families? Is conflict ignored so that it continues to fester and damage relationships, or is it managed openly and professionally in a healthy manner?

## Helping Mechanisms (Adequate Resources and Technology)

Do we have adequate equipment and technology to achieve the goals? Is our equipment in good working condition? Do we have policies, procedures, and processes that support achieving our goals? Do we have ample budget to achieve our goals?

## Outside Environment External Forces ("Everything Else")

What constraints and demands does the outside environment impose? How are outside forces influencing the organization? How does the global economy help or hinder achieving the mission and goals? Have government regulations affected our ability to achieve the mission? Are unions having an impact on the organization? In the case of health care, what external forces play a role with patients, their ability to pay for services, reimbursement for services from payers like insurance companies and the government? How has the Internet changed patients' access to medical information, and what effect does this have on medical practices? Who are the main competitors? Is there a parent organization that affects the organization?

Subsystems are in dynamic equilibrium. Change in any one subsystem has implications for the others. Every subsystem needs to be reexamined as they shift to ensure that they all still fit. For example, what are the implications if there is a shortage of resources and the income stream declines? What if conflict escalates among team members? What if some leadership members leave?

Careful monitoring of the subsystems is essential for ensuring that there is congruency among the subsystems. No subsystem can operate independently. If one subsystem changes, there will be changes in the others. For example, if there was a change in the relationships box in Exhibit 1.1 — reflecting a change in how conflict is managed among the team members — this change affects all the other internal subsystems and can strain the outside domains as well.

## EACH SUBSYSTEM DIRECTLY IMPACTS OTHERS

When constructing the subsystems, it is imperative to understand that each subsystem directly impacts the strength of the other subsystems. For example, if you want to develop a high-performing team approach, it is critical that all six boxes facilitate and foster team behavior. The leaders would commit to work as a team, model team behavior, and train others how to behave on a high-performing team. The mission statement and values would include teamwork. The reward and recognition system would reward team-building behaviors and provide discipline for selfish, solitary ones. The team member relationships would receive a lot of focus, and members would be taught conflict management techniques and communication and collaboration skills. The organization structure would discourage "silos" and foster teamwork. The mechanisms would include state-of-the-art equipment in good working condition in order to facilitate productive effort and working relationships.

## COMMUNICATING TO TEAM MEMBERS

It's through the six subsystems — purposes, leadership, rewards, structure, relationships, and mechanisms — that team members learn what is important and how they should perform. The leaders are responsible for ensuring that the messages the team receives are consistent and clear, and that they are focused on the customer as well as the vision, mission, and values. See Exhibit 1.2 for examples of the communications that come through loud and clear to team members.

| EXHIBIT 1.2 | Communications that Come through Loud and Clear to Team Members |
|---|---|

| | |
|---|---|
| Reward systems | The way people dress |
| Verbal language | Style of leadership |
| Body language | Letters to customers |
| Office layouts | Formal communication |
| Working conditions | Informal communication |
| Decision-making process | Website |
| Human resources policies | E-mails from leadership |
| Benefits | Treatment of customers |
| Professionalism of leaders | Respect displayed |
| Cues | Organizational structure |
| Process improvement systems | Work distribution |
| Working relationships | Conflict management |
| Signals and codes that come from leadership actions | Training/Development opportunities |
| Types of feedback given — coaching/disciplining | Where budget is spent |
| Promotions | Value hiring |
| Demotions | Values |
| Coaching, mentoring | Celebrations |
| On-boarding process | Press releases to community |
| Actions by leaders | |

© 2009 Susan A. Murphy, MBA, PhD

## CREATING AN ALIGNED AND CONGRUENT ORGANIZATION, ONE SUBSYSTEM AT A TIME

Asking the question "If it were perfect, what would this subsystem look like?" can be a very effective process for creating an aligned and congruent system. For example, If it were perfect, what would our mission be? If it were perfect, what would our leadership look like? What about our reward and recognition system? Our structure? Our relationships and how we manage conflict? Our helping mechanisms?

Throughout the chapters in this book, we'll be examining each of the subsystems, and we'll see that by strengthening each of the six boxes, we can strengthen the overall medical practice. See Exhibit 1.3 for the 6 box model in input/output terms.

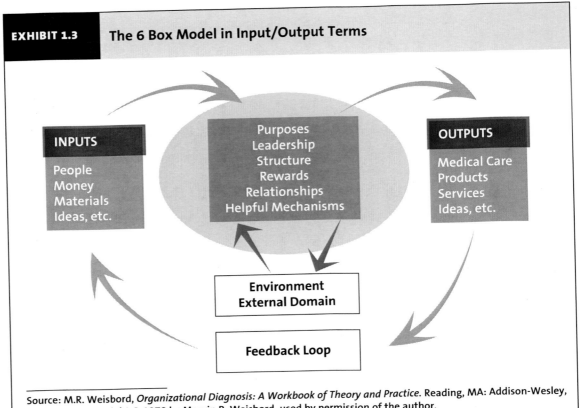

**EXHIBIT 1.3**    **The 6 Box Model in Input/Output Terms**

**INPUTS**

People
Money
Materials
Ideas, etc.

Purposes
Leadership
Structure
Rewards
Relationships
Helpful Mechanisms

**OUTPUTS**

Medical Care
Products
Services
Ideas, etc.

Environment
External Domain

Feedback Loop

Source: M.R. Weisbord, *Organizational Diagnosis: A Workbook of Theory and Practice*. Reading, MA: Addison-Wesley, 1983, p. 12. Copyright © 1978 by Marvin R. Weisbord, used by permission of the author.

## DIAGNOSING POTENTIAL EXTERNAL DISRUPTIONS

Another way to think about the six boxes is that each is continually being juggled to keep up with shifting — and uncertain — winds in the external domain, or as "everything else outside." These external domains include the following:

➤ Customers (patients, families, visitors);

➤ Suppliers (of materials, pharmaceuticals, capital, equipment, space);

➤ Competitors (for both markets and resources);

➤ Regulatory groups (government, unions, trade associations, certifying groups); and

➤ Parent organizations (university, central headquarters, corporate office).

So, as we're building and strengthening a medical practice, it helps to discover how the external domain is straining the internal subsystems (relationships, rewards, leadership, structure, etc.) as well as how the internal issues may be straining relations with one or more important external domains. See Exhibit 1.4 for a diagnostic tool to benchmark your team effectiveness.

| EXHIBIT 1.4 | Benchmarking Your Team Effectiveness |
| --- | --- |

### 20 CHARACTERISTICS OF HIGH-PERFORMING TEAMS

The 20 characteristics in this diagnostic tool are based on characteristics of high-performing teams. Distribute this questionnaire among your team members and have them complete it anonymously. The characteristics are in the Likert scale format to be scored 1 to 7, where 1 means this characteristic in not present in your team and 7 means it is very evident.

Collect the instrument from your team members and for each of the characteristics, calculate the mean score and the range. This will demonstrate where your organization is excelling and where you can focus on continuous improvement to increase your team's performance. The lower the mean score and the wider the range, the more attention the characteristic requires from you as the leader. The optimum scores are a high mean and narrow range.

### INSTRUCTIONS FOR EXERCISE

Indicate your assessment of your team and the way it functions by circling the corresponding number on a scale of 1 (low) to 7 (high).

Choose the number that you feel is most descriptive of your team.

### 1. MISSION/VISION/GOALS/PRIORITIES

(Low)  Team members don't know the mission/vision/goals/priorities.

(High)  Team members completely understand and agree with mission/vision/goals/priorities.

| 1 | 2 | 3 | 4 | 5 | 6 | 7 |

### 2. VALUES AND STANDARDS

(Low)  We have very different values, and our standards are not clear.

(High)  We all understand our values and standards and strive constantly to live up to them.

| 1 | 2 | 3 | 4 | 5 | 6 | 7 |

### 3. BRANDING

(Low)  We are not different from similar organizations; our reputation is not distinguishable.

(High)  Our brand is clear. Patients come to us because we're the best.

| 1 | 2 | 3 | 4 | 5 | 6 | 7 |

### 4. LEADERSHIP

(Low)  One person dominates, and leadership roles are not shared.

(High)  There is full participation in leadership; leadership roles are shared by members.

| 1 | 2 | 3 | 4 | 5 | 6 | 7 |

*(continued)*

**EXHIBIT 1.4**
*(continued)*

## Benchmarking Your Team Effectiveness

### 5. EMOTIONAL INTELLIGENCE

(Low)     Leaders do not practice self-management, self-control, or empathy.

(High)    Leaders practice self-management, self-control, and empathy.

| 1 | 2 | 3 | 4 | 5 | 6 | 7 |
|---|---|---|---|---|---|---|

### 6. LEADERSHIP COMMUNICATION

(Low)     We do not know what is going on in other parts of the organization.

(High)    We are informed about important issues within the organization.

| 1 | 2 | 3 | 4 | 5 | 6 | 7 |
|---|---|---|---|---|---|---|

### 7. STRUCTURE

(Low)     Our organizational structure is neither efficient nor effective.

(High)    Our organizational structure is efficient and effective.

| 1 | 2 | 3 | 4 | 5 | 6 | 7 |
|---|---|---|---|---|---|---|

### 8. TRAINED, PROFESSIONAL TEAM

(Low)     Staff is not oriented nor trained in their jobs.

(High)    Staff is oriented, well trained, and professional.

| 1 | 2 | 3 | 4 | 5 | 6 | 7 |
|---|---|---|---|---|---|---|

### 9. PERFORMANCE

(Low)     We can't get projects finished; we don't follow through on commitments.

(High)    We deliver on time, on budget, and follow through on commitments.

| 1 | 2 | 3 | 4 | 5 | 6 | 7 |
|---|---|---|---|---|---|---|

### 10. UTILIZATION OF RESOURCES

(Low)     Member resources are not recognized or used.

(High)    Member resources are fully recognized and used.

| 1 | 2 | 3 | 4 | 5 | 6 | 7 |
|---|---|---|---|---|---|---|

### 11. ROLES AND RESPONSIBILITIES

(Low)     Team members are unclear in their roles, responsibilities, and performance expectations.

(High)    There is clarity in job roles and responsibilities of team members.

| 1 | 2 | 3 | 4 | 5 | 6 | 7 |
|---|---|---|---|---|---|---|

### 12. REWARDS AND RECOGNITION

(Low)     Outstanding performance is neither recognized nor rewarded.

(High)    Outstanding performance is always recognized and rewarded.

| 1 | 2 | 3 | 4 | 5 | 6 | 7 |
|---|---|---|---|---|---|---|

### 13. TRUST AND CONFLICT

(Low)     There is little trust among members, and conflict is evident.

(High)    There is a high degree of trust among members. Conflict is dealt with openly and worked through.

| 1 | 2 | 3 | 4 | 5 | 6 | 7 |
|---|---|---|---|---|---|---|

### 14. COMMUNICATION/LISTENING

(Low)    We are guarded and cautious in team discussions, and we don't listen to each other.

(High)   We are open and authentic in team discussions, and we listen and feel understood.

1          2          3          4          5          6          7

### 15. DEGREE OF MUTUAL SUPPORT

(Low)    We operate on the basis of everyone for himself/herself.

(High)   We show genuine concern for each other.

1          2          3          4          5          6          7

### 16. DIVERSITY

(Low)    Prejudice exists among team members and differences are not appreciated or respected.

(High)   Differences among team members are respected and appreciated.

1          2          3          4          5          6          7

### 17. PROBLEM SOLVING/DECISION MAKING

(Low)    There is no consistent way that problems are solved or decisions are made.

(High)   Team has well-established and agreed-upon approaches to problem solving and decision making.

1          2          3          4          5          6          7

### 18. CONTROL AND PROCEDURES

(Low)    There is little control and a lack of procedures to guide team functioning.

(High)   There are effective procedures; team members support these procedures and regulate themselves.

1          2          3          4          5          6          7

### 19. INNOVATION/CHANGE/CREATIVITY

(Low)    The team is rigid and does not experiment with how things are done.

(High)   The team experiments with different ways of doing things and tries new ideas.

1          2          3          4          5          6          7

### 20. CELEBRATION

(Low)    Successes are not acknowledged or celebrated.

(High)   Team acknowledges and celebrates successes.

1          2          3          4          5          6          7

## Exercise    What Else Is Going On? Scanning "Everything Else"

How satisfactory do you view current transactions between these external domains and your medical practice?

|  | Highly Unsatisfactory |  |  |  | Highly Satisfactory |
|---|---|---|---|---|---|
| Patient/Family/Visitor | 1 | 2 | 3 | 4 | 5 |
| Supplier | 1 | 2 | 3 | 4 | 5 |
| Competitor | 1 | 2 | 3 | 4 | 5 |
| Regulator | 1 | 2 | 3 | 4 | 5 |
| Parent organization | 1 | 2 | 3 | 4 | 5 |

Do you have any influence over the situation?

_____

_____

NOTE: This exercise is also on the CD.

## Exercise    External Environment

List three important environmental demands that influence your practice's strategic mission (major purpose for existing).

1. _____

2. _____

3. _____

NOTE: This exercise is also on the CD.

## CHAPTER PRESCRIPTIONS

➤ Ensure that the leaders in your organization are aware of what's occurring externally (outside the organization) and become proactive leaders.

➤ Increase awareness by the managers as well as the team members about the subsystems and together work toward fulfilling the mission and values, leadership, rewards and recognition, structure, relationships, and helping mechanisms throughout the organization.

➤ Understand that each subsystem does not work independently of the other, but rather directly impacts the strength of the others.

# The Role of Compensation and Incentives in Engaging the Team ································

Laura Jacobs, MPH and Mary Witt, MSW
—*The Camden Group*

We all remember the oft-quoted phrase "Follow the money." This mantra is never more true than when it comes to translating organizational goals from words to desired behavior and outcomes. As the backbone of any medical practice, physicians set the tone for the culture and operating environment of the organization (the "system"), and engaging physicians in the process of strategic planning as well as establishing goals and performance expectations is critical. Just as critical, though, is translating those priorities into a compensation and incentive structure for physicians and staff that ensures the desired attributes and outcomes are appropriately rewarded.

This chapter explores the ways in which compensation systems can be structured to ensure that the financial (and other) incentives "fit" with the desired vision, strategies, and goals of the practice. Too often, physician compensation and incentives become the focus of attention because of a need to react to a negative influence: the need for a financial turnaround, competitive threats of physicians leaving the group, internal jealousies between physicians, and so forth. And even more frequently, physician compensation and incentives are designed in a vacuum, without regard to team member incentives. As discussed throughout this book, the inter-dependencies of the systems of the practice must be acknowledged and addressed to achieve success. And there's nothing more obvious than incentive systems to illustrate what the organization values. This includes the benefits that are offered. Increasingly, physicians are as interested in the "lifestyle" they can enjoy in the practice as they are in the income they will derive while practicing there.

Designing and implementing a compensation structure for physicians, though, is not for the faint-hearted. As described later in this chapter, the process of designing or modifying a compensation plan is nearly as important as the result, because the outcome must have the support and understanding of management and physicians. Although much has been and will continue to be written on compensation structures for physicians, this chapter focuses on the key elements of compensation design that support the engagement of all team members to jointly support the achievement of the medical practice's goals and desired culture.

## THE CONTEXT FOR PHYSICIAN COMPENSATION

It's important to frame the environment that influences physicians' outlooks and perspectives on compensation. For many years, as shown in the Exhibits 2.1 and 2.2, annual compensation increases have been less than the rate of productivity increase. That is, physicians are working harder, yet not necessarily reaping the benefits in terms of increases in income. This is a result of the simple fact that reimbursement increases are not keeping up with practice expense increases. Exhibit 2.3 illustrates the increasing proportion of dollars going to pay operating expenses, as indicated by the

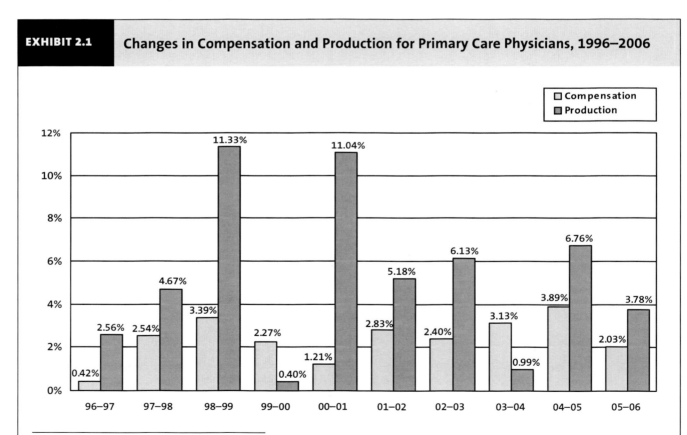

**EXHIBIT 2.1**  **Changes in Compensation and Production for Primary Care Physicians, 1996–2006**

Source: From the *Physician Compensation and Production Survey: 2007 Report Based on 2006 Data.* Reprinted with permission from the Medical Group Management Association, 104 Inverness Terrace East, Englewood, Colorado 80112. www.mgma.com. Copyright 2007. Page 20.

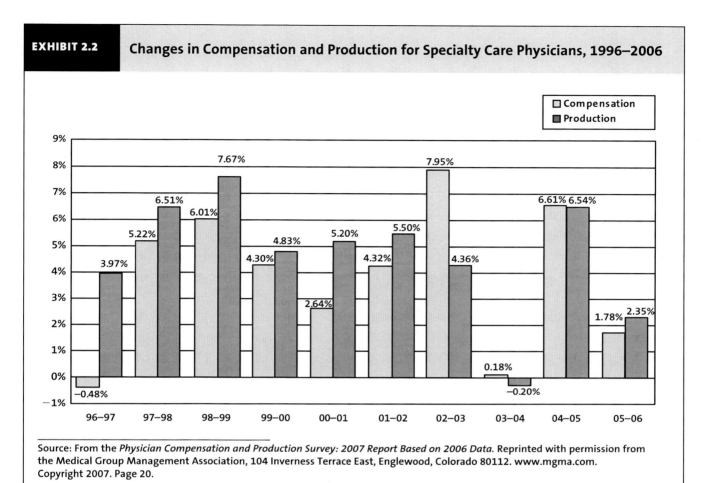

EXHIBIT 2.2 **Changes in Compensation and Production for Specialty Care Physicians, 1996–2006**

Source: From the *Physician Compensation and Production Survey: 2007 Report Based on 2006 Data.* Reprinted with permission from the Medical Group Management Association, 104 Inverness Terrace East, Englewood, Colorado 80112. www.mgma.com. Copyright 2007. Page 20.

Medical Group Management Association® (MGMA) surveys of multispecialty groups. This economic reality puts a strain on compensation systems, because there tends to be a shrinking pool of dollars available to pay physicians in the group. Studies indicate that primary care physician incomes declined, adjusted for inflation, by 10 percent between 1995 and 2003; surgical specialists' inflation-adjusted income dropped by 8 percent, and medical specialists' income merely kept pace with inflation.[1]

At the same time, we are facing a period where there are shortages of physicians emerging in many specialties. Particularly critical is the supply of primary care physicians, as shown in Exhibit 2.4. This trend puts pressure on compensation and benefits, because with demand exceeding supply, pure economics would indicate that compensation levels will increase. This is in direct conflict with the preceding point that there are fewer dollars available to pay physicians. So one can see why physician compensation discussions are about as appealing for most practice administrators as enduring a root canal.

| EXHIBIT 2.3 | Median Total Operating Costs as a Percent of Total Medical Revenue: 1990–2005 |

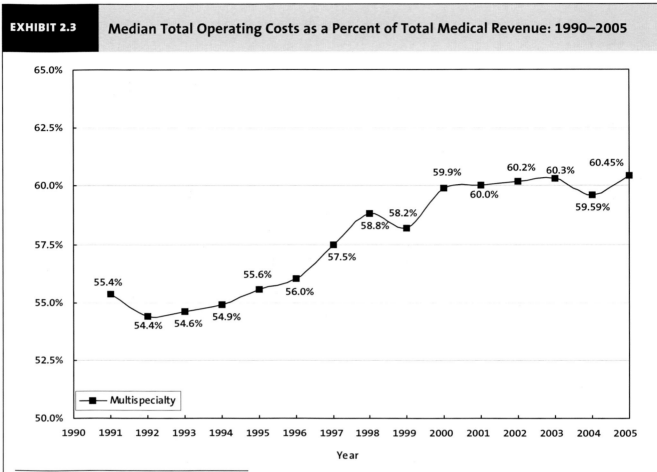

Source: From the *Cost Survey for Multispecialty Practices: 2006 Report Based on 2005 Data.* Reprinted with permission from the Medical Group Management Association, 104 Inverness Terrace East, Englewood, Colorado 80112. www.mgma.com. Copyright 2006. Page 16.

If this weren't difficult enough, the regulatory climate puts restrictions on how physicians can get paid, even within a medical group. The federal Stark regulations limit how physicians get paid for ancillary services (laboratory, radiology, durable medical equipment) production as well as putting strict guidelines in place for physicians employed or compensated by hospitals. Any compensation model, particularly one that is productivity based, must also be concerned with compliance with fraud and abuse regulations; there must be adequate protections in place to ensure that physicians are billing not only what is documented in the medical record but what is medically appropriate as well.

New on the horizon are pay-for-performance incentives being rolled out by payers. Some, like Medicare, are starting with so-called pay-for-reporting structures, which provide small incentives for providing data necessary to monitor quality and adherence to generally accepted protocols for managing patients. Many private payers are also providing either incentives for reporting or payment for better-than-average outcomes on a series of measures.

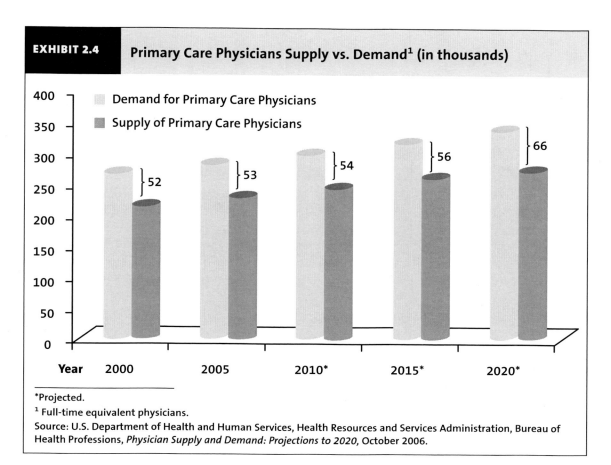

**EXHIBIT 2.4** — Primary Care Physicians Supply vs. Demand[1] (in thousands)

Demand for Primary Care Physicians
Supply of Primary Care Physicians

| Year | 2000 | 2005 | 2010* | 2015* | 2020* |
| --- | --- | --- | --- | --- | --- |
| Gap | 52 | 53 | 54 | 56 | 66 |

*Projected.
[1] Full-time equivalent physicians.
Source: U.S. Department of Health and Human Services, Health Resources and Services Administration, Bureau of Health Professions, *Physician Supply and Demand: Projections to 2020*, October 2006.

Despite the rudimentary nature of these pay-for-performance systems, it is generally accepted that they spell a trend for the future: "value-based purchasing." This means that payers and employers will pay more for superior performance on quality and other measures, and less for those providers (hospitals and physicians) who score below average. So, as much as physicians and others may argue over the appropriateness of the measures, the fact is that payments will increasingly depend on the performance of the practice on certain quality and patient satisfaction measures. For the purposes of designing a compensation plan, then, it will be important to introduce measures and incentives that match the reward structures established by payers. (Remember: "Follow the money.")

## WHAT PHYSICIANS WANT

Physicians want what all of us want: fair and reasonable compensation and a workplace that allows them to use their skills in the most effective way possible. They also want to be surrounded by colleagues who share a similar outlook and culture. But within those generalities, differences are emerging as the generation gap between Baby-Boomer and Generation-X physicians is demonstrated in work styles and expectations. The "I had to work my way to the top" outlook of Baby Boomers just doesn't compute with the Gen Xers.

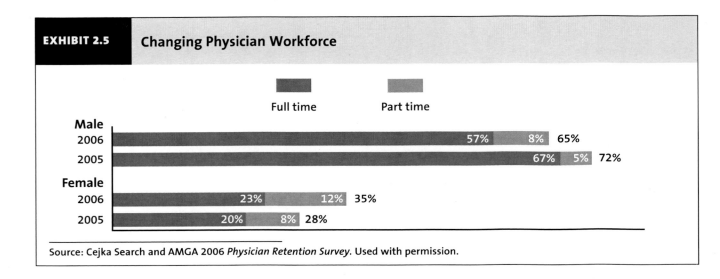

**EXHIBIT 2.5** | **Changing Physician Workforce**

Source: Cejka Search and AMGA 2006 *Physician Retention Survey*. Used with permission.

And the 60-plus-hour workweeks of the Baby Boomers don't mesh with the Gen Xers' need for work–family balance. These conflicts tend to come out in discussions about compensation: Gen Xers are interested in the paid-time-off policy, whereas the Baby Boomers are interested in the productivity formula.

Another demographic trend to be factored into compensation models is the growing percentage of female physicians. As shown in Exhibit 2.5, in one year alone, between 2005 and 2006, females have increased from 28 percent to 35 percent of the workforce in a recent survey conducted by the American Medical Group Association (AMGA) and Cejka Search. This survey also showed that 20 percent of all physician employees work part time, of which 60 percent are female. Also notable, however, is that for both males and females, the percentage working part time increased during this period. This trend is expected to continue, as the proportion of new medical school graduates who are female has risen to 50 percent.[2] Therefore, compensation structures that allow for part-time physicians will be a necessity, if they aren't already.

Although compensation often gets a lot of attention as a reason for physician dissatisfaction or turnover, the AMGA/Cejka Search survey indicates that other nonmonetary reasons frequently drive turnover. The most oft-cited reason for voluntary resignations was "poor cultural fit with the practice," followed by "relocated to be closer to family" (see Exhibit 2.6). This speaks to the need to watch all aspects of the practice environment, not just compensation. Exhibit 2.7 reinforces this point, with survey results regarding effective retention strategies. "Regular feedback and performance reviews," "partnership/ownership opportunities," and "flexible work hours or part-time options" were the three most important activities impacting physician retention. We will cover the importance of feedback later in this chapter.

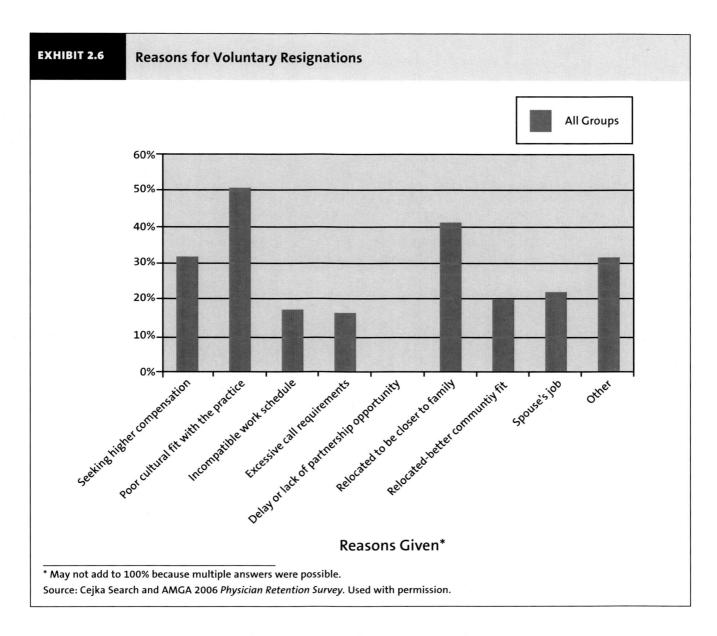

**EXHIBIT 2.6**   **Reasons for Voluntary Resignations**

All Groups

Reasons Given*

* May not add to 100% because multiple answers were possible.
Source: Cejka Search and AMGA 2006 *Physician Retention Survey*. Used with permission.

The important point in this discussion is that a group's compensation plan must take into consideration the expectations of the current and potential recruits to the practice. This means weighing all key issues such as the balance of benefits and cash, flexibility in work hours, feedback mechanisms, partnership track, as well as the degree to which compensation is "incentive driven."

## WHAT ELSE INFLUENCES COMPENSATION DESIGN?

We have discussed the general trends that are impacting not only compensation design but physician perspectives on compensation. But there are many other factors to consider when designing a compensation plan. Exhibit 2.8 illustrates some of these factors.

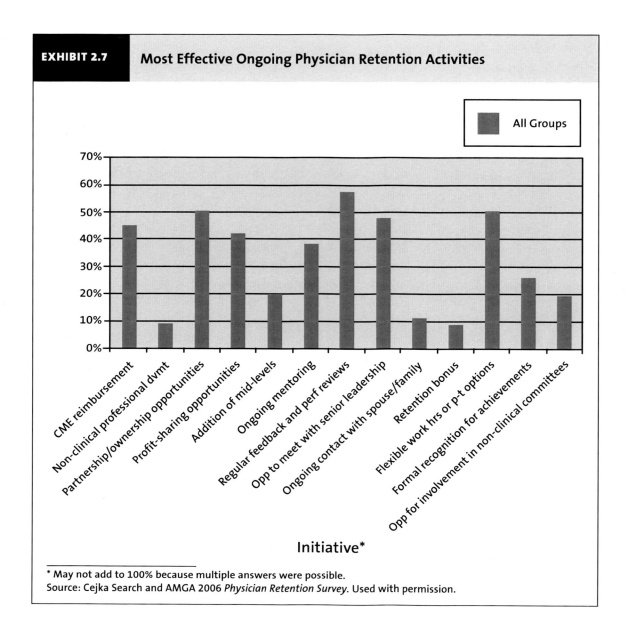

**EXHIBIT 2.7** | **Most Effective Ongoing Physician Retention Activities**

* May not add to 100% because multiple answers were possible.
Source: Cejka Search and AMGA 2006 *Physician Retention Survey*. Used with permission.

## Internal Factors

The most important factors on the list in Exhibit 2.8 are (1) financial position and (2) strategic objectives. Why? The financial position of the group will influence the amount of compensation that must be incentivized. If the group is stable, it may be okay to have a high percentage of compensation driven by set salaries, with incentives driven by a profit pool. On the other hand, a group that must turn around financial performance must put greater pressure on physicians to engage in the turnaround, meaning that a greater proportion of the compensation should be driven by factors that will affect financial performance, such as productivity and expense management.

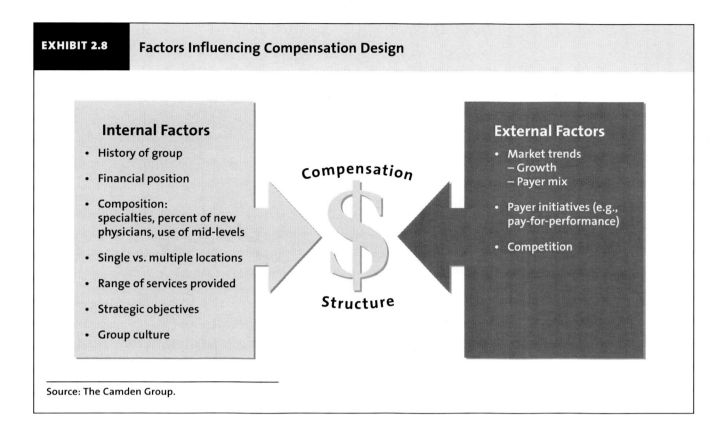

**EXHIBIT 2.8** | **Factors Influencing Compensation Design**

**Internal Factors**
- History of group
- Financial position
- Composition: specialties, percent of new physicians, use of mid-levels
- Single vs. multiple locations
- Range of services provided
- Strategic objectives
- Group culture

**Compensation** **$** **Structure**

**External Factors**
- Market trends
  – Growth
  – Payer mix
- Payer initiatives (e.g., pay-for-performance)
- Competition

Source: The Camden Group.

The strategic objectives of the group are the starting point for setting the goals of the compensation plan. How does the group wish to reposition itself for the future? By increasing patient volume; changing payer mix; improving quality or patient service; providing new services or expanding into new markets? Are there operational goals or cultural goals that require change in physician behavior? The size and composition of the group is next in importance — what works for a small, single-specialty group is not likely to work for a larger multispecialty group.

## External Factors

Also to be considered are market factors that influence both the competition for physicians as well as the structure of reimbursement to physician groups. For example, if there are many large groups in the market that offer a rich benefit package (pension, vacation, etc.), even small groups will have to think about how to structure their compensation package to provide a competitive alternative. If payers in the region are beginning to structure pay-for-performance incentives, then the group must consider how to motivate individual physicians to achieve top performance within the measures used by payers. (Did we say, "Follow the money?")

## WHAT INCENTIVES ARE THE RIGHT INCENTIVES?

The first question should be ... "How much of the physician's compensation should be 'at risk'?" That is, how much is base (or fixed) salary vs. variable? The smaller the group, the more variable compensation tends to be, because the group will merely split the net income (collections minus office expenses) among the physicians in the group according to a predetermined formula. Larger groups tend to set a base salary, to be adjusted by the various incentives (productivity, collections, expense management, quality, etc.); this comprises the variable compensation. We avoid the use of the word *bonus,* because all of the compensation is for work completed; the variable portion is just more sensitive to actual performance. At a minimum, variable compensation should comprise no less than 10 percent of total cash compensation (excluding benefits). Anything less than 10 percent is "of interest," which can get physicians' attention to monitor performance but isn't likely to truly drive change.

Next, the question is, "What should we measure and tie to compensation?" Exhibit 2.9 provides some examples of measures that help to achieve selected strategic objectives.

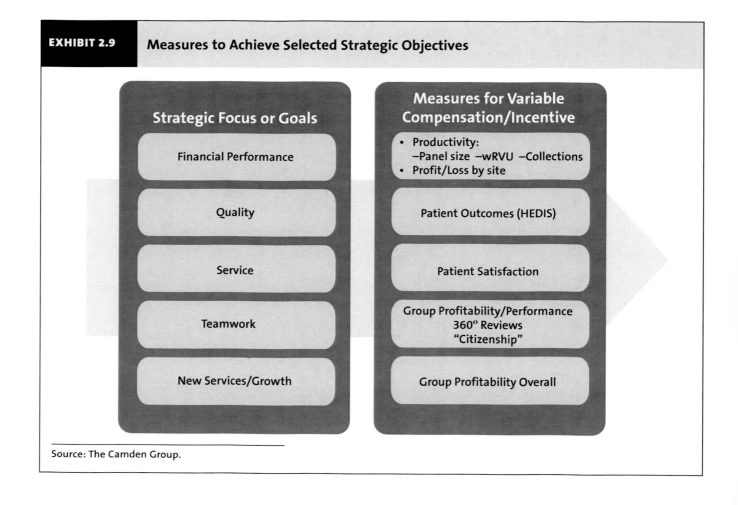

**EXHIBIT 2.9**   **Measures to Achieve Selected Strategic Objectives**

**Strategic Focus or Goals**

Financial Performance

Quality

Service

Teamwork

New Services/Growth

**Measures for Variable Compensation/Incentive**

- Productivity:
  −Panel size −wRVU −Collections
- Profit/Loss by site

Patient Outcomes (HEDIS)

Patient Satisfaction

Group Profitability/Performance
360° Reviews
"Citizenship"

Group Profitability Overall

Source: The Camden Group.

The following case studies provide some illustrations of how the compensation structure fits the strategic position and goals of the medical group. We've also provided a brief analysis of the advantages and disadvantages of each model.

## The Egalitarians Model

This group is a four-person cardiology group that has existed for 20-plus years. The last person to join the group joined five years ago. The egalitarians group grew from a two-person practice and includes physicians that provide a variety of cardiac services — two are interventional cardiologists and two are noninvasive cardiologists. Members of the egalitarians decided long ago that it was important to bring in physicians with a variety of talents, but that the whole group should benefit by the multidisciplinary nature of the practice. That is, just because the invasive cardiologist might benefit from higher reimbursement from the procedures s/he performs, it is because the physician is in a group that allows him/her to concentrate on those procedures. This group highly values teamwork and the "all for one and one for all" mentality. As a small group, there is visibility on the productivity of each member, so it was never a concern that physicians might not "hold their own." The advantages and disadvantages of this model are presented in Exhibit 2.10.

## Individual Accountability Model

This multispecialty medical group is composed of 40 physicians, predominately primary care, but has approximately 10 specialists. They operate in a partially managed care environment and have been primarily salary-based for most of their 15-year history. They want to increase physician accountability and, at the same time, ensure that the medical group excels in pay-for-performance programs that local payers are rolling out. Here's how they designed their plan:

- Base salary: 80 percent of market rate.
- Incentive pay: Pool driven by group profitability. Incentives paid based on individual performance in:
  - Productivity: measured by weighted panel size (health-maintenance-organization and fee-for-service patients) as well as work relative value units (wRVUs);

---

**EXHIBIT 2.10  Advantages and Disadvantages of the Egalitarians Model**

| Advantages | Disadvantages |
|---|---|
| - Promotes teamwork<br>- Promotes focus on overall group profitability and positioning | - Difficult to allow for part-time physicians (or partial retirement)<br>- Doesn't work as well in larger groups |

| EXHIBIT 2.11 | Advantages and Disadvantages of the Individual Accountability Model |
| --- | --- |

| Advantages | Disadvantages |
| --- | --- |
| ➤ Provides a range of incentives that match the goals of the group — from individual productivity to quality and patient service. The fact that the indicators are measured is often a driver for performance, regardless of the amount of money at risk. | ➤ Requires good measurement tools and reporting structures for feedback. |
| ➤ The overall pool is driven by the group's profitability, which helps to promote a group focus on performance. | ➤ A relatively small amount of money is at risk for quality and service performance, which could be interpreted that these are not really "valued" by the group. |

- Patient satisfaction: measured by access (third next available appointment); continuity (degree to which primary care physicians see their own patients); and patient surveys; and
- Quality/Teamwork: HEDIS (Health Plan Employer Data and Information Set) scores; staff and peer satisfaction (360-degree surveys); medical record reviews.

Productivity measures account for 80 percent of the incentive, with patient satisfaction and quality/teamwork each at risk for 10 percent. The group believes that over time, a greater share of the incentive will go to the service and quality measures as the pay-for-performance programs from payers increase their potential payments. Exhibit 2.11 notes the advantages and disadvantages of this model.

## Focus on Finance Model

This multisite, single-specialty group has had recent financial troubles and is concerned about engaging its physicians in the financial turnaround. It has put in place a compensation program that mirrors how the physician would function as if s/he were in private practice. Collections are allocated to the physician who performed the work, and expenses are allocated depending on whether they are fixed, variable, or individual. For example, rent and administrative costs are distributed equally among each of the physicians; supply costs are variable; individual expenses, including extra staffing, are charged to the individual physician. Exhibit 2.12 outlines the advantages and disadvantages of this model.

| EXHIBIT 2.12 | Advantages and Disadvantages of the Focus on Finance Model |
| --- | --- |

| Advantages | Disadvantages |
| --- | --- |
| ➤ Physicians become very engaged in managing both the revenue stream and expenses of their practice.<br><br>➤ Fairly allocates expenses where they are used. | ➤ Can create competition within the group; does not promote teamwork.<br><br>➤ The focus on individuality can lead to a breakdown in group initiatives — physicians are not likely to want to go to a new location, particularly if the payer mix is not as attractive. |

As these case study examples show, there are almost as many ways to design compensation programs as there are medical groups. The important thing to remember is to match your group's situation and goals with the drivers of the compensation plan; wherever there's a mismatch, you're likely to be frustrated with the results. Did we mention, "Follow the money"?

## DRIVING EXCELLENCE — SETTING EXPECTATIONS

Extraordinary medical practices are not afraid to set expectations and measure performance. As discussed earlier in this book, excellence starts with a vision that drives organizational objectives and performance targets. Without clearly defined performance targets at all levels of the organization, it becomes difficult, if not impossible, to create an approach to compensation that appropriately aligns incentives with the organization's mission and vision. Exhibit 2.13 illustrates the relationships among vision, organizational objectives, performance targets, and compensation.

Physicians are highly goal-directed, as demonstrated by their years in medical school and residency, so clearly articulated goals and performance standards help them focus their energies and activities to achieve success. Because physicians place high value on autonomy and independence,[3] it is important to involve them in the setting of the performance targets to achieve buy-in. Performance standards should be based on a set of criteria that defines the responsibilities and expectations. Exhibit 2.14 displays the qualities of effective expectations.

Of course, creating a performance target is not sufficient in and of itself to drive performance. It is critical that targets are routinely measured to monitor progress, positive or negative variances are identified, and action plans to

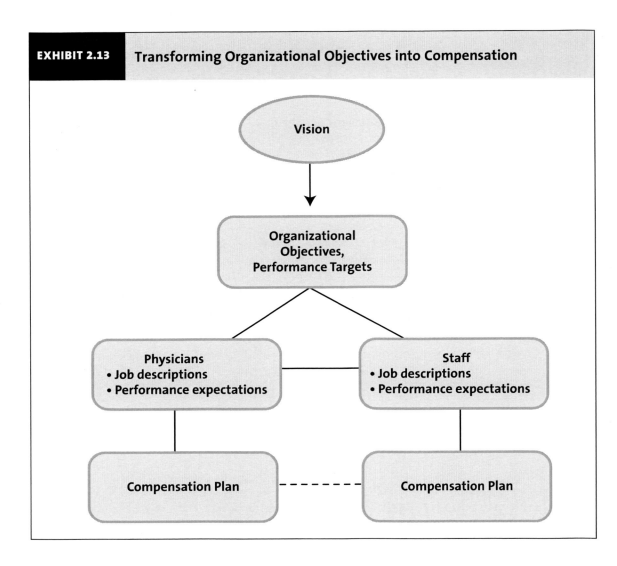

**EXHIBIT 2.13** | Transforming Organizational Objectives into Compensation

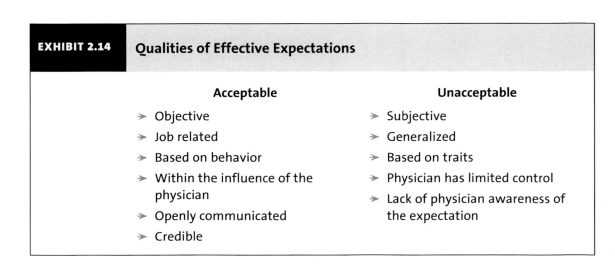

**EXHIBIT 2.14** | Qualities of Effective Expectations

| Acceptable | Unacceptable |
|---|---|
| ➤ Objective | ➤ Subjective |
| ➤ Job related | ➤ Generalized |
| ➤ Based on behavior | ➤ Based on traits |
| ➤ Within the influence of the physician | ➤ Physician has limited control |
| ➤ Openly communicated | ➤ Lack of physician awareness of the expectation |
| ➤ Credible | |

address negative variances are quickly implemented. As already stated, feedback is an important physician satisfier, so they should receive regular feedback about their success in meeting targets.

Feedback on performance targets can and should be provided through a variety of approaches. Monthly physician dashboard reports inform physicians of their individual performance and also can show them how they compare to other physicians within the organization.

Because physicians are highly influenced by data, the use of dashboard reports can be a particularly effective way to gain physician attention. Physicians highly value the respect of their peers, so sharing of the data among all physicians can be an effective method for motivating physicians to improve their performance as compared to others. We believe that transparency is key here — sharing the names of physicians and their performance is better than blinded results. That way, physicians with less-than-average performance can seek the advice of the top performers, or at least observe what they might be doing differently.

Regular group and one-on-one meetings also aid in monitoring and reinforcing physician performance. Group meetings provide a forum to publicly recognize those physicians who have gone above and beyond, as well as to review organizational performance against targets, especially the physician dashboard report. It also provides an opportunity to engage the physicians in brainstorming and discussion about critical medical group issues. Moreover, these meetings provide a venue in which to strengthen physician knowledge through education.

One-on-one meetings provide an opportunity to provide feedback, discuss problem areas, and solve problems. In addition, they ensure that physicians have an opportunity to provide their feedback and input to physician leadership. These meetings are an effective vehicle by which to mentor and coach new physicians. Meeting frequency should be determined by the amount of time the physician has been with the medical group, their practice maturity, and performance. For young physicians, those new to the medical group, or those with performance issues, meetings should occur at least monthly. If there are performance issues, a weekly schedule may provide a better opportunity to monitor progress and ensure compliance. Quarterly meetings with established physicians may be sufficient. If scheduled meetings are infrequent, it is incumbent on physician leadership to provide other opportunities to communicate so that physicians can share their issues and concerns as well as be updated on the activities of the medical group as a whole.

Clear expectations provide direction to physicians, establish a mechanism to create accountability within the organization, and provide a marker for management to assess the contribution made by the individual to the success of the organization. The following example demonstrates how clearly defined expectations can assist both the physician and the organization in achieving their goals.

## Case Study: Use of Performance Targets

Johnstown Medical Group recruited a new physician, Dr. George, and his practice had grown much more slowly than anticipated. During the recruitment process, the medical group emphasized that Dr. George would have to actively market his practice in order to maintain his income level after his salary guarantee ended, but there was no discussion about specific expectations. At six months, Dr. George felt frustrated, misled, and unsupported, while the medical group felt that Dr. George wasn't meeting expectations because he hadn't done the marketing they expected.

If the medical group had identified specific performance measures, Dr. George would have had clear direction on how he was to market and what the medical group expected from him. At the same time, the medical group would have had measurable standards with which to hold Dr. George accountable. Unfortunately, instead, they were left to argue about what was meant by "marketing."

In order to resolve the issue, the medical group and Dr. George agreed to mutually identify specific performance expectations related to marketing. The specific expectations identified were:

- Dr. George will schedule at least one luncheon per week with potential referring physicians.
- Dr. George will speak at least monthly at a community service organization, school, employer, or other group in venues that provide opportunities to introduce himself to the community. The medical group will provide Dr. George with a list of organizations to contact regarding speaking engagements.
- Dr. George will join one service organization and become an active participant.
- Dr. George will contact the local newspaper and offer to write a monthly column. If the offer is accepted, the administrator will interview Dr. George on the topic of the column and do the actual writing.
- The administrator and Dr. George will meet weekly to review progress. Dr. George will meet with the lead physician monthly.

Dr. George now had a clearly defined road map to guide his marketing efforts, and he knew what support he could expect from the medical group in this effort. The medical group had a set of measurements by which to assess Dr. George's performance. A mechanism to monitor (weekly and monthly meetings) and discuss performance was implemented. These meetings provided a forum in which both parties could hold the other accountable for achieving the growth required to sustain the practice. As a result of defining expectations and behavior for both parties, Dr. George succeeded in achieving the required growth target within two months of the original target date.

# FORMAL PERFORMANCE EVALUATION

Formal performance measurement is critical to the success of any organization. As Jim Collins states in his book *Good to Great*,[4] great organizations make sure they have the right people on the bus in the right positions. Unless specific individual performance standards have been created and a formal process to evaluate performance exists, it becomes difficult to identify and address getting the right people on and off the bus.

Performance targets, dashboard reports, and regular meetings to provide feedback on performance are key components of a formal evaluation process. The additional elements include use of an evaluation tool and a formal meeting between physician and supervisor for review of and feedback on performance.

In creating an evaluation tool, it is beneficial to include a self-evaluation section, thereby providing the opportunity for the physician to provide input into the formal evaluation. Use of a self-evaluation portion can provide an effective vehicle by which to identify specific physician "motivators," explore opportunities for integrating the physician's personal goals with organizational objectives, and to problem-solve areas that need improvement. It also can provide a reality check to measure the congruence of the assessment by the individual with that of others.

In addition to self-evaluation, the evaluation tool should include quantitative data on productivity, patient relations/satisfaction, quality (patient outcomes), efficiency (resource utilization), dependability, and teamwork. The physician dashboard report can, and should, provide the basis for this section of the evaluation tool.

Many organizations also have added a component called the 360-degree evaluation. The 360-degree evaluation is a multi-rater approach whereby physicians and staff who frequently work with the physician are asked to provide feedback on the physician's performance. The purpose of this tool is to measure the physician's strengths in working with others to care for patients and meet organizational objectives. Those completing the evaluation could include other physicians in his/her call group, other clinical providers such as nurse practitioners and physician assistants, his/her medical assistant, front office staff, and/or medical group management. In using this tool, it is important that evaluators are only asked to evaluate those traits or criteria with which they have personal experience. The rating system should be easily understood, and careful instruction should be given to evaluators on how to apply the rating system in order to achieve consistency of application.

The meeting for the formal performance review provides an opportunity to review the past year and to plan for the upcoming year. It should build on data and feedback that has been provided to the physician during the past year. There should be no surprises. These meetings can facilitate collaboration, enhance communication, and establish mutually acceptable goals and performance targets for the year to come.

## PHYSICIAN LEADERSHIP AND ACCOUNTABILITY

Organizational and physician excellence is impossible to achieve without effective physician leadership. Successful physician leaders articulate a vision, create a culture of accountability, instill confidence, and effectively manage change. They translate vision into performance targets, they recognize the need to continually monitor progress in achieving those targets, and they don't hesitate to address failures in accountability.

As critical as the role of the physician leader is, medical groups often have difficulty in determining whether they have the right physician leaders in place because they lack the tools to evaluate performance. Physician leadership effectiveness is tied to the leader's ability to effectively relate to and communicate with the physicians, management, and staff within the medical group. It is important to evaluate leadership performance as well as that of individual physicians, but medical groups are often reluctant to address leadership inadequacies, thereby seriously handicapping the medical group as it tries to enhance success. Exhibit 2.15 provides a simple tool to assess the performance of your medical group leaders. The 360-degree tool can be a particularly valuable approach to assessing leadership performance since it involves a variety of constituencies.

## NONMONETARY INCENTIVES

In reviewing physician values and what they want from work, it quickly becomes clear that compensation is only one component of what they are seeking from work. As the AMGA/Cejka Search survey made clear, although competitive pay is a must in this era of physician shortages, compensation alone rarely attracts, motivates, or retains physicians.

Physicians and other team members evaluate their relationship with their work by comparing what they give at work (time, work effort, loyalty) to what

| EXHIBIT 2.15 | How Do You Know You Have the Right Leader? | Consistently No | | | Consistently Yes | |
|---|---|---|---|---|---|---|
| | | 1 | 2 | 3 | 4 | 5 |
| 1. | The leader is skilled at influencing others and promoting an idea or vision. | ☐ | ☐ | ☐ | ☐ | ☐ |
| 2. | The leader is readily available and approachable. | ☐ | ☐ | ☐ | ☐ | ☐ |
| 3. | The leader is good at varying his/her approach based on the situation. | ☐ | ☐ | ☐ | ☐ | ☐ |
| 4. | The leader listens carefully to the medical group's physicians, management, and staff. | ☐ | ☐ | ☐ | ☐ | ☐ |
| 5. | The leader is willing to accept different viewpoints. | ☐ | ☐ | ☐ | ☐ | ☐ |
| 6. | The leader confronts others skillfully and tactfully. | ☐ | ☐ | ☐ | ☐ | ☐ |
| 7. | The leader works actively to problem solve rather than blame. | ☐ | ☐ | ☐ | ☐ | ☐ |
| 8. | The leader has the ability to persuade while maintaining a collaborative relationship. | ☐ | ☐ | ☐ | ☐ | ☐ |
| 9. | The leader accepts feedback and responds well to feedback. | ☐ | ☐ | ☐ | ☐ | ☐ |
| 10. | The leader is decisive. | ☐ | ☐ | ☐ | ☐ | ☐ |

Source: The Camden Group.

they receive (pay, recognition, sense of accomplishment). Today's younger physicians seek a practice lifestyle that allows for life outside of the practice, and most are coming into practice with large debts from medical school. Older physicians may be more focused on productivity, retirement benefits, and recognition for their years of service. All generations want recognition for their contributions as well as the opportunity to influence decisions.

In response to these needs, medical groups are continually reexamining their recruitment packages, benefit structures, physician scheduling, partnership/ownership options, and governance. Recruitment packages may include income and practice expense guarantees, student loan repayment, signing bonuses, and, in some cases, housing loans.

Physician benefits routinely average between 12 percent and 17 percent of their cash compensation.[5] Benefits generally include health and disability insurance, retirement, and paid time off. Physician time off averages approximately six weeks per year for vacation and continuing medical education. More medical groups are exploring the feasibility of offering deferred compensation plans to address the needs of those older physicians concerned about retirement.

Physician work and call schedules are more likely to become a point for negotiation as physicians seek to limit their work hours and improve their quality of life. As more women become physicians, the demand for part-time schedules has increased. Medical groups are struggling to find innovative ways to meet these demands while ensuring patient care and minimizing the financial impact of the medical group. Solutions include:

- Flexible scheduling, that is, expansion of clinic hours to allow for morning or evening shifts; this approach also has the added benefit of meeting the needs of the working patient.
- Practice job sharing whereby two physicians or a physician and clinician (nurse practitioner, physician assistant) share a practice.
- Increased use of nurse practitioners and physician assistants to provide "first call" to limit disruptions to personal life when on call.
- Hiring of hospitalists to assume care for those patients requiring hospitalization.

There can be an inherent tension as physicians join groups and struggle to maintain the autonomy and independence they have always valued. Therefore, medical groups may want to identify decisions at the local individual practice level where physicians can exercise some autonomy and independence of judgment within parameters established by the medical group governance structure.

The ability to achieve partnership/shareholder status also influences physician satisfaction. Younger physicians are less willing to tolerate partnership/shareholder tracks that exceed three years. At the same time, new physicians often lack the capital to pay large amounts to become medical group owners. Consequently, medical groups often spread the purchase price (if there is one) over several years to address this issue.

## HOW DO WE REDESIGN COMPENSATION?

Autocratic or dictatorial compensation redesign is rarely successful—in fact, many administrators have found it to be a lethal "career-limiting" move. Instead, successful redesign should be a team effort, but team members cannot be just anyone. It generally is not helpful to include all of the physicians in the organization unless the organization is small. It also should be a physician-led initiative and should begin with the medical group governing body. Although administrative staff can support the redesign process, physicians must drive the process in order to create credibility for the process and facilitate physician buy-in.

| EXHIBIT 2.16 | **Checklist for a Compensation Check-up** | | | |
|---|---|---|---|---|

|  | No | Sort of | Yes |
|---|:---:|:---:|:---:|
|  | 1 | 2 | 3 |
| 1. We conduct a market comparison of physician compensation, including benefits, annually. | ☐ | ☐ | ☐ |
| 2. Our physician compensation is generally competitive with market norms for cash compensation and benefits. | ☐ | ☐ | ☐ |
| 3. Most physicians could describe how our incentives are calculated. | ☐ | ☐ | ☐ |
| 4. Physicians are provided feedback on a variety of performance measures regularly (for example, monthly productivity, annual patient satisfaction). | ☐ | ☐ | ☐ |
| 5. Our physician incentives are aligned with our organizational goals, strategic priorities, and culture. | ☐ | ☐ | ☐ |
| 6. Our physician incentives are aligned with the performance goals of our management team and staff members. | ☐ | ☐ | ☐ |
| 7. Our physician compensation structure is aligned with our sources of revenue (payer mix, pay-for-performance initiatives). | ☐ | ☐ | ☐ |
| 8. Our compensation structure makes allowances for flexible work hours (for example, part-time or flexible hours). | ☐ | ☐ | ☐ |
| 9. Once the incentives and total compensation are calculated, the variances between physicians seem appropriate, given performance, specialty, or other considerations. | ☐ | ☐ | ☐ |
| 10. Our leadership group has reviewed the overall compensation structure and its fit with internal and external factors within the last 18 months. | ☐ | ☐ | ☐ |

Source: The Camden Group.

Before beginning redesign, it is important to understand the efficacy of the existing compensation plan. The assessment of your current plan should begin by examining how it contributes to organizational success. By asking key questions, you can determine if physician and medical group incentives are aligned and answer whether the plan is driving successful performance on those factors critical to the success of the organization. Exhibit 2.16 provides a quick diagnostic tool to help start this evaluation.

An effective compensation redesign team starts with the medical group's governing body and may include a compensation committee. The governing body should set the direction for compensation redesign based on organizational and financial goals. In larger groups, it should also make the final decision regarding the compensation plan, whereas smaller groups will more likely rely on unanimous consent. Exhibit 2.17 illustrates the role of governance, management, and physicians in the redesign process.

**EXHIBIT 2.17**     **Roles in Compensation Redesign**

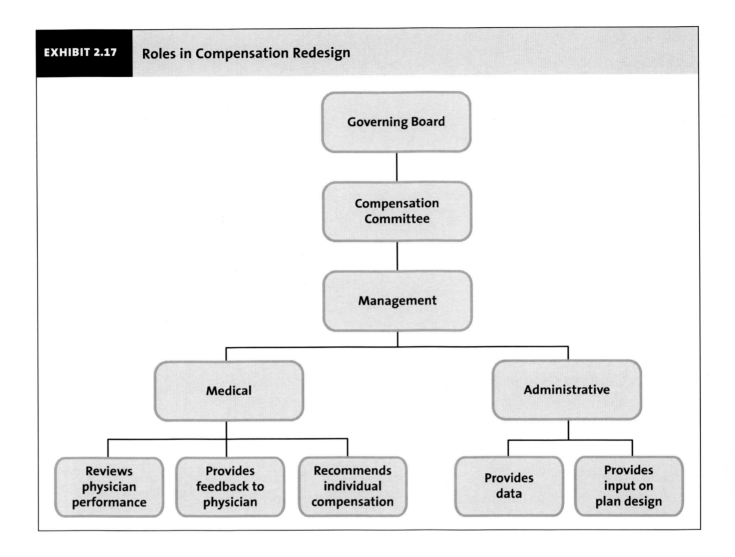

The governing body may wish to create a compensation committee to perform the detailed work of compensation redesign as well as to regularly monitor the plan's effectiveness. This committee would discuss and review potential options and their impact on the medical group. Based on direction from the governing body, it can make recommendations regarding the compensation methodology and identify the potential outcomes. The committee should be representative of the various physician constituencies such as specialties and/or clinical sites to ensure that various viewpoints are considered in the decision-making process. At the same time, it is important to the credibility of the process that representatives be perceived as acting without self-interest; that is, their primary obligation should be to the welfare of the medical group as a whole rather than to their own interests. Management representation is also key, to ensure that the mechanisms exist to regularly measure and report the data necessary for incentives and related measures.

# COMMUNICATION, COMMUNICATION, COMMUNICATION

Compensation redesign often creates high physician anxiety, so frequent communication during the process is a must in order to manage physician concerns and expectations. The governing body can agree on a well-designed compensation methodology and still have the compensation plan fail because the plan was not appropriately communicated.

Communication of the process and the plan must begin with the governing body. It should introduce the redesign process as it begins and provide updates as the process moves toward completion. After it approves the plan, the governing body should present it to all physicians by clearly explaining the rationale for redesign and placing the new methodology in the context of how it supports success in achieving organizational goals. Individual leaders, such as the medical director, site medical directors, department chairs, and compensation committee members, should then be responsible for meeting with each physician to discuss the plan's potential impact on each individual.

It is helpful to model compensation by physician under the new methodology in order to address individual physician concerns about how it will impact them, but those discussions have to occur within the framework of organizational requirements. If the redesign is a significant change in methodology, the medical group may wish to run a "shadow" plan for several months before implementation to allow physicians to adjust to the new approach. Of course, this assumes that the medical group is not in a financial crisis and can implement the new plan over time.

It is important to remember, however, that effective medical groups do not stop communicating when compensation redesign is completed. Successful medical groups develop ways to solicit regular physician input and feedback. Physician surveys, opportunities to participate in governance and decision making, as well as group and one-on-one physician meetings provide opportunities to solicit physician advice and input.

# PROMOTING PHYSICIAN–STAFF TEAMWORK

Physicians do not work in a vacuum. Without staff support, it is unlikely that productivity targets can be met — staff behavior impacts physician efficiency, and patients judge their satisfaction with care by their interactions with staff as well as with physicians. Therefore, organizational goals, performance targets, and compensation must reinforce physician–staff teamwork.

Staff job descriptions should reflect their roles in ensuring timely patient throughput and volume, creating patient satisfaction, managing expenses, and facilitating physician efficiency. Physician job descriptions should acknowledge their role as a team member. It is useful to have a code of conduct that addresses treatment of others; timeliness and tardiness standards need to be consistently applied to both physicians and staff, because inconsistent applicability of performance standards can lead to conflict and legal challenges.

## Managing the Human Resources Component

Optimizing teamwork between physicians and staff often introduces a human resources component, so clarity of roles, responsibilities, and reporting relationships is a necessity. Although physicians have a role to play in providing feedback about staff job requirements and performance, their role is generally not that of supervisor. Physicians can create or magnify problems with staff when they attempt to intercede. It is not unusual for staff to attempt to play the physician against the supervisor to get what s/he wants when they sense that there is disunity between the supervisor and the physician. Exhibit 2.18 delineates the difference between the role of management and the physician team member as it relates to staff.

## Linking Financial Incentives

As medical groups strive to increase physician efficiency and manage operating expenses, they are often linking physician and staff compensation through the creation of incentive programs based on practice profitability. Under such arrangements, both physicians and staff receive variable compensation if profitability targets are met. However, it is weighted differently based on the ability of each to impact the profitability targets.

| **EXHIBIT 2.18** | **Management and Physician Team Member Roles as Related to Staff** |
|---|---|
| **Management** | **Physician** |
| ➤ Develops staff job descriptions and performance standards | ➤ Provides input into staff job descriptions and performance standards |
| ➤ Provides direction on nonclinical tasks | ➤ Provides direction on clinical tasks |
| ➤ Supervises staff job performance | ➤ Provides feedback on staff job performance |
| ➤ Determines staff compensation | ➤ Provides input on staff compensation merit increases |

As with physician compensation, if the group wishes to structure performance incentive compensation for team members, the expectations for performance must be clear at the outset. Even if there isn't a staff bonus structure, letting the staff know how physician compensation is structured — at least what the performance measures are — will allow staff to support physician achievement.

Some medical groups have focused on targets in specific areas; for example, volume, operating expense, and/or patient satisfaction targets. With the advent of pay-for-performance, medical groups also are considering ways to reward both physicians and staff for achieving quality goals. When linking incentives between staff and physicians, it is important to clearly delineate the roles and responsibilities as well as the ability to influence the outcome to ensure proper recognition and rewards for specified behaviors. Incentives can quickly become disincentives if any party is penalized or held accountable for items outside of their responsibility or control.

In linking incentives, it is important to recognize that physicians and staff play different roles in achieving organizational targets, and their impact or influence on specific targets may be significantly different. So although the target may be the same, clarity on how the outcome can be impacted by individual performance must be communicated to each team member, based on his/her roles and responsibilities. For example, one metric that could drive variable compensation for both staff and physicians is patient satisfaction. And although both staff and physicians influence response time to patient requests or phone calls, their responsibilities vary, and their locus of control over the outcome also differs. The receptionist is responsible for quickly answering a patient's call, taking an accurate message, and giving it to the physician, although the physician must return the call. Both could be rewarded for contributing to achieving expectations for patient satisfaction, but there must be individualized communication about how each can impact the result.

## SUMMARY

As described here, the process, structure, and implementation of compensation plans is a critical link to facilitating the achievement of the medical practice's goals. It is a fundamental component to keeping the "system" working as one — all oars pulling in the same direction. The incentives and other components that drive the compensation structure are a telling sign of what the group's leadership truly values. Despite what may be written in the strategic plan, if the strategic priorities don't translate into evidence as illustrated in the workplace structure, monetary incentives, benefits, team objectives, or individual performance measures — all efforts to craft a meaningful direction for the medical group — will be in vain. Remember, "Follow the money."

## CHAPTER PRESCRIPTIONS

➤ Evaluate your group's compensation plan for both physicians and staff. Do its design and incentives support your organizational goals?

➤ Set performance targets for physicians and provide them with regular feedback on how their actual performance compares to the targets. Consider using monthly "dashboard" reports.

➤ Use formal performance evaluation tools for physicians just as you would with staff. They need feedback from medical leaders on how to improve performance; otherwise you're limiting your potential to reach your group's goals.

➤ Assure staff that performance expectations support the goals you have set for physicians. This includes supporting practice growth, profitability, and patient satisfaction, or other targets that have been set for overall group performance.

## REFERENCES

[1] Center for Studying Health System Change, *Tracking Report.* Results from the Community Tracking Study, No. 17, June 2007.

[2] U.S. Department of Health and Human Services, Health Resources and Services Administration, Bureau of Health Professions, *Physician Supply and Demand: Projections to 2020,* October 2006.

[3] A. Sheldon, *Managing Doctors* (New York: Aspen Publishers, 1986).

[4] J.C. Collins, *Good to Great* (New York: HarperBusiness, 2001).

[5] MGMA Cost Survey: 2006 Report Based on 2005 Data for Single Specialty Practices.

Contributing authors **Laura Jacobs, MPH,** is senior vice president and **Mary Witt, MSW,** a vice president at The Camden Group in El Segundo, California. For more than 20 years, Ms. Witt and Ms. Jacobs have each led strategic development, compensation redesign, and operational performance improvement of medical groups across the country.

## CHAPTER 3

# Interviewing and Hiring····························

Jim Collins, author of the best-selling book
*Good to Great,*[1] found that great companies: (1) Get the right people on the
bus; (2) Get the right people in the right seats; (3) Get the wrong people off
the bus; and (4) Put who before what.

## THE RIGHT PEOPLE ON THE BUS AND IN THE RIGHT SEATS

Great companies have rigorous selection processes for getting new people on
the bus. They invest substantial time in evaluating each candidate, making
systematic use of at least three evaluation devices, for example, interviews,
references, examination of background, meeting members of the family, test-
ing. "When in doubt, we do not bring the person on the bus ..."

## NEVER, EVER RUSH!

Never rush into a hiring decision! Sure, that position's been open a long
time, and you're worn out from pulling weekends and late evenings trying to
keep it all together. However, putting the wrong person in the wrong job can
make things even worse — and for a long, long time.

There are important benefits for making good hiring decisions. One of the
primary reasons is that you can strengthen the culture you're creating by
screening and hiring someone who emulates the values and behaviors in
which you believe. The people whom you hire and the people whom you fire
communicate clearly to your team the values which you believe are important. By making good hiring decisions, you will have fewer staff performance
problems, fewer interruptions in workflow, and can elevate your organization
closer to the lofty vision you and your team have developed. Good hiring
decisions reduce the high costs of turnover. Replacing a staff member can
cost 50 percent to 150 percent of his/her annual salary in recruitment and
orientation costs for the new staff member. And that doesn't include the

potential loss in continuity and quality in your organization, stress to the rest of the team while they cover the vacant position, and the time you spend screening and interviewing other candidates.

## FIRST THINGS FIRST

What is the first thing to do when you have a vacant position? Determine whether the vacancy needs to be filled. If so, with what kind of skill set? One of the temptations that we have is to immediately start looking for someone like the person being replaced. Look at the job from a fresh point of view. This could be an opportunity to restructure, reorganize, or promote. If you need to replace the position, do you need the same type of position? On the CD, there is a case study example from Providence Health & Services of a workflow chart that the organization made to examine the flow of a patient through their system. Making the chart to review work-flow resulted in the decision to change the assignments and add a position with a different skill set in order to more efficiently, effectively, and profitably streamline the operations.

## DEFINE THE JOB

What is the purpose of the job? What is the ultimate product or service that the person in this position needs to perform? What is the relationship of this job to others in the organization?

What will this new team member do? What are the most important duties that this new team member will perform? What is the nature and scope of his/her decision making?

How will this new team member perform the job? What are the reporting relationships? What are the general working conditions? That is, what are the hours and days of the week? Where will the person report? Who are the coworkers/peers of this team member?

Are special interpersonal skills required? Does this person interact with patients frequently? What specific skills and training are needed for this new position? Is it important that this person be detail oriented? What skills are absolutely necessary?

What about physical attributes? Is physical strength required? Is size a factor? If you elect not to hire a disabled person, you must be able to show specifically how the disability prevents the person from doing the work. I have included information about the Americans with Disabilities Act on the CD.

# WRITE THE JOB DESCRIPTION

Define the qualifications necessary to fill the job. Include the correct duties, responsibilities, qualifications, licenses, and/or certifications. Verify the job title and salary range. Attach the rules of conduct to the job description if you've decided to include the behaviors from the rules of conduct in the job description. I believe that introducing the rules of conduct as a part of the interview/screening process is an important way to inculcate the behaviors that you want into your organization. Determine the technical, self-management, and team dimensions of the job.

# INTERVIEWING GUIDELINES

By following certain guidelines, you can ensure successful hiring practices (see Exhibit 3.1). Taking time to prepare prior to the interview and adhering to consistent interview practices, you can make hiring more efficient and help to promote selection of a candidate who will be qualified, perform well, and fit well with your team, your values, and your culture.

| EXHIBIT 3.1 | Review Resume in Light of Qualifications Necessary | | |
|---|---|---|---|
| | | Assess | Comment |
| Determine if job candidate's resume provides evidence of meeting the technical and self-management dimensions of job. | | | |
| Look for job accomplishments. | | | |
| Beware of qualifiers: "knowledge of," "assisted with," "exposed to." | | | |
| Don't excuse sloppiness (typos, errors in punctuation, and spelling). | | | |
| Look for red flags: too many jobs in recent years, unclear indication of leaving jobs. | | | |
| Remember that people often get help with their resumes; the resume may not be indicative of candidate's true communication skills. | | | |

NOTE: This exhibit also appears on the CD.

# TELEPHONE INTERVIEW PREQUALIFICATION

Time is a precious commodity, so consider prescreening via a telephone interview. Exhibit 3.2 provides a sample interview process.

| **EXHIBIT 3.2** | **Telephone Interview Screening** |
| --- | --- |

Candidate: _____ Date: _____

Interviewer: _____

**INTRODUCTION**

Hello, my name is _____ from _____. I received your application for the position of _____ in the _____ Department. Are you still interested in this position? I am conducting telephone interviews, so is this a good time to discuss your skills and qualifications for this position? This interview will take about 15 minutes. If not, can we schedule a different time to discuss your background?

**QUESTIONS**

Why are you looking to leave your current position? What interests you in this position? What is your current salary? _____ What are your salary expectations? _____

**(As the manager, it's important to note what the salary range is for this position.)**

Please tell me about your previous work experience. What skills and abilities do you have that you feel qualify you for this position?

What does *excellent* customer service mean to you? Can you give me an example of a time when you provided excellent customer service in the past six months?

The work hours for the position are _____, and you are expected to be at work on time. Can you meet this job requirement?

There may be times when overtime is necessary. Are you able to meet this job requirement?

Do you have any questions about the position?

**CLOSING**

At this point, you should determine whether the candidate is interested, qualified, available, and willing to interview further for the position.

If the candidate's salary requirements are not within your range and budget, you can let him/her know what the salary range is and determine their level of interest. If the salary range is not acceptable, thank him/her for the interview. If there is interest by you and the candidate for an interview, briefly explain the next steps.

*(Sample)*

*Thank you for taking the time to discuss your skills and background with me. I plan to finish telephone interviews by (date) and will then be selecting candidates for a personal interview. I will contact you directly if you are selected to participate in the next steps in this process. Is this the best number to reach you? Thank you for your time, and for your interest in _____.*

Source: University of California, Irvine Medical Center. Used with permission.

## CHOOSE INTERVIEW TEAM

Select who will be interviewing the candidate. Depending on the nature of the position, it may be wise to have the candidate interview with you, team members in the same department (to provide a better indication of the daily work and environment), and, if it is a supervisory position, any future staff the person would have. In higher-level positions, members of management should be included, and often the interviews should consist of several group interviews, to include different levels of staff.

It is best to meet with these groups beforehand to go over who should be asking which questions or covering certain topics and to ensure that they ask department-specific questions. Explain what is expected of the interviewing team as far as feedback after the interviews; make sure you stress documentation of the candidate's responses. Develop some core questions prepared as a basis for comparison.

Decide what kind of interview you'd like to conduct — straight questions and answers, role playing, or scenarios after which you ask the candidate how they would respond. Many organizations are utilizing behavioral interviewing techniques to get to know more about the candidate, how the person will work with the other team members, treat customers, and so forth. Exhibit 3.3 lists questions to avoid during an interview.

## PREPARE FOR THE INTERVIEW

Choose an appropriate environment for the interview — one where there will be privacy and no interruptions. When scheduling candidates, allow time between candidates so that you can take notes after each interview. Confirm the interview by sending an e-mail to the candidate with the following information:

> ➤ Location and time of the interview;
> ➤ Names of the interview committee, if applicable;
> ➤ Copy of the job description; and
> ➤ Copy of the rules of conduct.

## CONDUCT THE INTERVIEW

*Sweaty Palms* is the title of a book about interviewing. Although I've never read the book, I've always liked the title because it's descriptive of almost every interview I've ever conducted. And I've conducted more than 4,000 interviews. Some candidates spill coffee, trip, and faint. Others do just fine. Others learn about themselves by answering reflective questions about their values, skills, and goals that they had never considered.

| EXHIBIT 3.3 | Questions to Be Avoided | |
|---|---|---|
| **TOPIC** | **WHAT CAN'T YOU ASK?** | **WHAT CAN YOU ASK?** |
| **Age** | How old are you?<br>What is your birth date?<br>What year did you graduate? | Are you over 18? |
| **Citizenship/<br>National Origin** | Are you a U.S. citizen?<br>Where were you born? Where were your parents born?<br>What is your native language? | Are you authorized to work in the United States? [not necessary to ask this — this is verified with the I-9 at time of hire].<br>What language(s) do you read/write fluently? (only if required by the position) |
| **Marital/Family Status** | Are you married?<br>Do you plan to have a family?<br>Do you have any children?<br>What are your child care arrangements? | Would you be able and willing to travel as needed for the job? (only if required by the position)<br>This position requires occasional overtime (nights and/or weekends); would this present a problem? Would you be willing to relocate if necessary?<br>*Note*: These questions should be asked of ALL applicants. |
| **Affiliations** | What clubs or social organizations do you belong to? | List any professional or trade organizations you consider relevant to the position. |
| **Personal** | How much do you weigh?<br>How tall are you? | Are you able to lift a 60-lb weight, as this type of physical activity is part of the job? [when specifically required in duties of job] |
| **Disabilities** | Do you have any disabilities?<br>Do you have any medical conditions?<br>Do you need accommodations to perform this job? | Are you able to perform the essential functions of this job, with or without an accommodation? |
| **Arrest Record** | Have you ever been arrested? | At time of offer, advise the candidate that the offer is contingent on completion of a clean criminal background check. |
| **Military Record** | If you were in the military, were you honorably discharged? | In what branch of the armed services did you serve?<br>What type of training did you receive in the military? |
| **Religion** | What religious holidays do you observe?<br>Does your religion prohibit you from working any particular days? | There are no legal questions related to this subject. |

NOTE: This exhibit also appears on the CD.

Create as comfortable an interview setting as you can; this should not feel like an interrogation. The more comfortable we make it for the candidates, the better chance we have of finding the best candidates for the job. We don't want to hire people who are the best at "interviewing." We want to hire people who are high performers in the job and will "fit" with the culture you are creating.

Be on time and avoid sitting behind the desk during the interview. Begin by coming out of your office to greet the candidate, introduce yourself, and shake hands. It can be very intimidating for a candidate to be led into an office where the interviewer sits waiting behind the desk. If you need to use your office, be sure that your calls are held or that your phone is forwarded to voice mail to prevent interruptions from calls. Sit close to the candidate, preferably at an angle. Be aware of glare on the candidate; avoid having the candidate facing a window. Offer the candidate a cup of coffee, water, or a cold drink.

Open the conversation with "icebreakers" to build rapport and make the applicant feel more at ease. Build a friendly atmosphere, show genuine interest, and listen attentively. Comment on the weather, ask about the traffic, compliment the candidate or interviewee on his/her suit, or if he or she found parking easily, and so forth. Many interviewers start with the question "Tell me a little about yourself," and candidates often start to ramble and get more nervous (unless they've taken interviewing courses). I recommend that you steer away from that type of question at the beginning.

Start your session with a brief overview of the position. Don't go into great detail, because that can sway their responses or limit them. The purpose of giving them a brief introduction is in case they misunderstood a major part of the job (such as required travel or occasional overtime), so that they have an opportunity to speak up before wasting your time and theirs.

## TALK LITTLE, LISTEN MUCH

Approximately 75 percent of the interview should be the candidate's responses to your questions. Managers should talk only 25 percent during the interview. Many inexperienced managers make a huge mistake when they talk 75 percent of the time rather than 25 percent. They don't get to know the candidate. Interview the candidate first and then, if s/he is still qualified and interested, describe more about the organization and position. I know of many managers who describe the culture that they want and then have the candidate describe the environment they are seeking. Such interviews go like this:

Manager: "We're looking for team players, who have positive attitudes, put patients first, and go the extra mile. What environment are you looking for?"

The candidate responds: "One where I can be a team player, display my positive attitude, put patients first, and go the extra mile!"

| EXHIBIT 3.4 | Sample Interview Questions from UCI Medical Center | | | |
|---|---|---|---|---|
| **Attributes** | **Questions** | **Least Desirable Answer** | **Most Desirable Answer** | **Rating** |
| **Opening Question** | Please tell us about your skills, abilities (and/or education) that you feel make you qualified for this position. | • States has no special skills or abilities, no education or experience<br>• States has applied for many different positions and has not been hired<br>• "I just need a job" | Describes in detail specific skills, abilities, education, and experience suitable to position. In addition, observe for:<br>• Interpersonal skills<br>• Team player<br>• Strong background<br>• Adaptability<br>• Good communication skills | ☐ Insufficient<br>☐ Adequate<br>☐ Superior |
| **Purpose** | Why are you interested in employment with us? | Provides answers such as:<br>• To get a job<br>• To work close to home<br>• Good benefits<br>• Need a change<br>• More money | Describes specifics related to:<br>• Great work environment<br>• Opportunity to advance<br>• Looking for new challenges<br>May mention:<br>• Good reputation<br>• Teaching facility<br>• Educational opportunities | ☐ Insufficient<br>☐ Adequate<br>☐ Superior |
| **Department-Specific Questions**<br>*(Please identify 5 questions — a scenario of a specific situation, as well as specific questions related to the exact skill set needed.)* | | | DEPARTMENT-SPECIFIC QUESTIONS:<br>_____<br>_____<br>_____<br>_____<br>_____<br>_____ | ☐ Insufficient<br>☐ Adequate<br>☐ Superior |

The goal of the interview is to get to know the person, their personality, behavioral characteristics, and unique competencies that will make them the right match for the job and your organizational culture.

During the interview process, you want to discern the following information about the candidate. The best predictor of future performance is past performance. So, find out the extent of their experience and effectiveness of past performance as it relates to your job requirements as well as their:

| Attributes | Questions | Least Desirable Answer | Most Desirable Answer | Rating |
|---|---|---|---|---|
| Customer Service | Describe the most difficult customer you ever had to assist? *(Prompt questions)* • How did you handle? • What was the outcome? • Would you do anything differently next time? | Answers: • Never had difficult customer • Informed supervisor • Blames customer | Describes specific examples w/o criticism or blame. Describes appropriate behaviors and verbal responses: • Takes ownership of problem • Is not judgmental of customer • Uses "I" statements • Articulates positive outcome | ☐ Insufficient ☐ Adequate ☐ Superior |
| Teamwork | What type of work environment do you prefer? | Unable to answer, or answers: • "Everyone does their own job" • "A boss that leaves me alone" • "No one bothers me" | Describes specific examples/behaviors such as: • Team oriented • Supportive environment • Involved • Respectful • Professional • Availability of resources/ training • Good communication | ☐ Insufficient ☐ Adequate ☐ Superior |

Source: University of California, Irvine Medical Center. Used with permission.

➤ Level of responsibility previously held (Is it the same? Less? More?);

➤ Skill level and knowledge level;

➤ Strengths and shortcomings (Would s/he help or hurt team performance?);

➤ Level of stability and maturity;

➤ "Fit" with your organizational culture; and

➤ Attitude and behavior toward customers, peers, management, and work load.

Ask open-ended questions. Don't ask questions that require a "yes" or "no," or short response. Asking open-ended questions allows the applicant to respond completely and often reveals more information that will lead into additional questions.

Exhibit 3.4 gives sample interview questions.

## Categories for Open-Ended Questions

Ask questions in categories such as:

1. **Past or current positions** — What did you enjoy most about your last job? How have your previous jobs prepared you for more responsibility?

2. **Relationships with people** — How would you describe your supervisor? How would you characterize your coworkers? What kind of people do you enjoy working with? What kind do you find difficult?

3. **Stimulating self-assessment** — What do you consider your greatest strength professionally? In what areas would you most like to improve? Why?

4. **Career aspirations** — What position do you expect to hold five years from now? What are you doing to achieve your career goals?

5. **Job application** — How can you apply your skills and experience to this position?

### *Questions for Physicians*

➤ **Commitment** — What do you like about being a physician? What do you dislike? What are your career aspirations?

➤ **Compassion** — What experiences have been most powerful in shaping your professional identity? What feedback have you been given about the first impression you make with patients and families? Describe some of the ways you establish rapport with patients and family members. Describe a conflict situation you have had to address with a patient. Describe a conflict situation you have had to address with your colleagues.

➤ **Skills** — Describe your skills as a physician. What is an example of a challenging patient and what skills did the situation require?

➤ **Charting/Record-keeping** — What record-keeping methods do you prefer? How do you feel about charting and keeping records up to date?

## Nonverbal Cues

Be sure to watch for nonverbal signals that the candidate is sending. Is his/her body language open, natural, and nondefensive? Is there good eye contact? Can you sense enthusiasm for the job? Does the person become tense when you ask about the reason for leaving his/her last position? If you feel that a candidate is hiding something when responding, ask the individual to elaborate in order to get more information or clarification.

## DESCRIBE THE ENVIRONMENT

After you've concluded that you'd like to consider this candidate, describe the vision, mission, and values of the organization. Let the person know what behaviors you expect from members of the team. Also, include any negatives about the position because creating too "rosy" an image does not give the applicant a true description of the position. During the hiring process it can be a good time for managers and other team members to strengthen their vision and mission statements.

## CLOSE THE INTERVIEW

Although it may be tempting to offer the position during the interview, don't do it. It's important to compare notes from this candidate with information gathered during the interviews with other candidates. Give the candidate an estimated schedule for the decision-making process, and let him or her know when you'd like the successful candidate to start working at your organization.

## CHECK REFERENCES

In screening the candidate's references, consider the following areas and ask relevant questions:

- ➤ Describe the organization's culture, values, and goals. Then ask, "Is this candidate aligned with these values and goals?"
- ➤ Explain the job. Then ask, "How do you think s/he would fit into the position?"
- ➤ If appropriate, ask, "When did s/he work for you? What were the job responsibilities?"
- ➤ Ask how they would describe the applicant's:
  - Attendance;
  - Dependability;
  - Skill level;
  - Level of discretion/confidentiality/good judgment;
  - Accuracy;
  - Team skills;
  - Customer service;
  - Strengths; and
  - Areas for improvement.
- ➤ "Why did candidate leave his/her position?"
- ➤ "Would you rehire this individual?" Yes_____ No_____
  If no, ask "Why not?"

End the conversation by thanking them for their time and cooperation.

## MAKE THE DECISION

As Jim Collins emphasizes in the book *Good to Great,* "put the who before the what."[1] Skills can improve, but personality and motivation will not change. J.W. Marriott, the founder of Marriott International, believes we're either born with motivation or we're not. It's something you can't usually acquire along the way. One of your candidates may have better skills, but it's important to consider all factors that can affect your workplace culture and goals.

Organizations that are known for their quality and effectiveness usually have a robust process for hiring and promoting their team members. In the late 1990s, Southwest Airlines had about 200,000 applicants per year, interviewed 35,000 and hired 4,000. The interviews are done not by human resources professionals, but by peers; that is, pilots hire pilots, reservations people hire people who make reservations.

Southwest has a People Department that identified 35 top pilots, then interviewed them to identify traits that the 35 had in common. Team skills were identified as very important for the pilots, so Southwest now probes candidates for concrete examples of their teamwork, and listens for warning signs like candidates who say "I" all the time. Southwest interviewers turned down a pilot with outstanding flying credentials because he was rude to a Southwest receptionist during the recruiting process.

Herb Kelleher, former chief executive officer of Southwest, says, "We draft great attitudes. If you don't have a good attitude, we don't want you, no matter how skilled you are. We can change skill levels through training. We can't change attitude."[2]

One big mistake I often witness in hiring is that managers tend to like and hire candidates who have personality styles similar to their own. Be aware of this — and focus on the position requirements and the skills and experience of the candidates. As tempting as it is to compare the candidate with yourself or with the incumbent, fight the urge. Every successful new hire who is a high performer, goal oriented, and fits with your culture enhances the ability to align team member performance with organizational goals.

## CHAPTER PRESCRIPTIONS

➤ Hiring new team members shouldn't be an opportunity to "replace" the previous employee. Think about how the new team member can fully serve the practice in the best ways possible.

➤ Make your vision and mission the main focus when advertising for a new position.

➤ Don't just "interview" a candidate, but find out whether s/he is truly a good fit for the organization. What can the new person bring to the practice that might be lacking?

➤ Use the hiring process to your advantage. Get to know the individual's true goals, and determine whether the candidate is a good match for the organizational goals you use to guide your practice.

## REFERENCES

[1] J.C. Collins, *Good to Great* (New York: HarperBusiness, 2001).

[2] J. Magretta and N. Stone, *What Management Is* (New York: Cahners Business Information, 2002) 207.

## CHAPTER 4

# Orientation ·················································

## Orientation is often dis-orientation. I wonder
how many new team members are spinning at the end of the first day with
their new employer.

New team members start the day excited, apprehensive, curious, enthusiastic,
hopeful, confident, insecure, cautious — the emotions are all over the map.
Will they like it? Will they succeed? Will they be accepted? How long will they
work there? As described in chapter 3 "Leading Through Change" in *Leading,
Coaching, and Mentoring the Team* (Book 2 in the Maximizing Performance
Management Series) about leading during times of change, the first stage of any
change is resistance, even for a positive change like a new job. An interesting
effect of the resistance stage is that we aren't able to listen well — and one of
the things we do to new hires is *talk at them,* sometimes for two days!

Change is a shift from the known to the unknown, and a new job means all
new territory. New hires need to adjust before we can become fully productive
again. The most frequent complaints about new team member orientation are
that it's overwhelming, boring, or that the new team member feels all alone to
sink or swim. I know many staff members who say their supervisors were on
vacation when they started working at a new job — these new hires floated
around aimlessly for a week until the supervisor returned. As the saying goes,
"You only have one chance to make a good first impression," and many organizations miss that opportunity. The result is often a "dis-oriented" team member
who is not productive, feels helpless, "goal-less," and is likely to leave within the
first 90 days. From my experience, more than one-fourth of staff members leave
within the first 90 days, and many return to their previous employer — if that
employer will take them back. This damages the new hire's self-esteem; costs the
organization large amounts of money in advertising, interviewing, and orientation; plus, there are hidden costs of wear and tear on staff morale as it spends
time and energy trying to get the new hire up to speed.

## PURPOSES OF A GOOD ORIENTATION PROCESS

Orientation is an important component of the recruitment and retention
process. It's not just a "meet and greet" activity, but a process with many

benefits. Some of the benefits from creating a comprehensive, well-planned new hire orientation include:

> **Reduced anxiety.** As mentioned at the beginning of this chapter, there are many emotions involved with starting a new job. A good orientation program helps reduce the anxiety that comes from entering the unfamiliar organization, provides guidelines for standards of conduct, and shows team members how they fit into the organization. When oriented well, the team member doesn't spend a lot of time trying to second-guess the role and responsibilities that are involved in the new position.

> **Reduced start-up costs.** A proper orientation can help the team member get up to speed and fully productive more quickly. This reduces the costs involved with learning a new job.

> **Reduced turnover.** As mentioned earlier, more than 25 percent of new hires leave within the initial three months of starting a new job. A poor orientation program often causes new hires to feel that they aren't valued very highly and that they are being set up to fail. Orientation demonstrates to staff members that they are valued and that the organization wants to provide them with tools to succeed in their new job.

> **Time saver for the manager.** The better the initial orientation, the less likely it is for the manager and team members to invest time later answering basic questions or correcting errors the new hire made because of not understanding some organization policies, procedures, or goals.

> **Realistic job expectations, positive attitudes, and job satisfaction.** It's extremely important that new team members learn as quickly as possible what the organizational goals and expectations are, what their roles and responsibilities are, how they fit into the organization, what they can expect from others in the organization, as well as the values and attitudes of the organization.

## WHY ORIENTATION PROGRAMS FAIL

There are several reasons orientation programs fail. The most significant causes are:

> The program is poorly planned;

> The new team member does not receive a clear picture of his/her role and responsibilities; and

> The new employee does not feel welcomed by the team.

Why is it so important for the new hire to feel welcome? When new team members feel welcome and accepted, they are more willing to ask questions, problem-solve, participate in making decisions, and take initiative. They become a productive member of the workforce much more quickly.

A comprehensive orientation program takes time, energy, commitment, and a monetary investment. However, it can pay off tenfold in benefits for the new hire, the department, and the organization.

## TIPS FOR A SUCCESSFUL ORIENTATION

Following are some tips to provide a successful orientation for new team members.

> **Examine your program from the viewpoint of the new team member.** Ask new team members what they want to know. Ask recent new hires what they wish they had learned at the start, plus what they liked and disliked about their orientation process. Because it will still be fresh in their minds, they can provide important input. Ask the senior management team what they want the new recruits to know about their jobs and the organization.

> **Start the orientation process as soon as the individual accepts the position.** Send an agenda with the offer letter that shows what time to start work, where to park, and where to present themselves on the first day. Keep in touch with the new hire from the time s/he accepts the offer until the time orientation begins.

> **Be ready for new team members.** Greet them; make sure a work area has been created for them on Day 1. Inform the other team members of the start date for the new hire and encourage them to reach out to him/her. Introduce the new hire to others in the office, and make them feel welcome.

> **Include the mission, vision, values, rules of conduct, history, and "who's who" at the orientation** to provide firm footing for new team members.

> **Answer the most fundamental questions of the new hire — how the work that s/he does impacts the department and the organization.** Allow enough time for each new team member to understand the roles of everyone in the department, and how his or her role fits into the big picture. Define the what, when, where, and why of the new position before expecting him or her to be fully productive — but don't overwhelm this new recruit, who is trying to absorb so many things at one time.

> **Anticipate questions from the new hires.** Provide them with answers to frequently asked questions, a glossary of the organization acronyms and buzzwords, a phone list, and an organizational chart that shows key positions. Distribute a list of company resources that includes the name and e-mail of people who are designated to answer questions.

> ➤ **Provide a departmental mentor or buddy to the new recruit for at least 90 days to assist with questions during the orientation process.** The mentor can provide a departmental tour and introduce the new team member to his/her coworkers. Choose the mentor carefully — select a positive and knowledgeable team member who is a good representative of your culture. Also, ensure that the mentor is able to commit time and energy to the new hire — if a mentor is working toward a strict deadline on an important project, save that mentor for another new hire after the demanding project is finished.

> ➤ **Make sure the new hire does not eat alone during the first week.** The first day is a good time for the manager to take the new team member to lunch and include other team members.

> ➤ **Create a positive experience for new hires so they will return home at the end of the day, eager to report to their families what a great opportunity they have at this new organization.** Help them feel eager about returning on the second day!

A successful orientation happens only if your new team member decides s/he has made a wise decision to join your organization.

Getting to know the other team members is an important step for having the new team member feel valued and cared for in the job. One company has bagels every Friday for the office, and whenever there's a new hire, the bagels are served at his/her desk. Before team members can take a bagel, they must introduce themselves to the new hire. It's been a delicious way to welcome new team members on board.

Some organizations list new members in the newsletter. Others create a team member book that has pictures of each member and some information that each wants to share with the others. These can include interests, hobbies, family, favorite type of music, favorite food, favorite movie, favorite book, role with the organization, and so forth. New team members are immediately included in the team member book. Some organizations send the information via e-mail as an announcement and a welcome. Another puts the new team member's name on the marquis. I smile as I remember accepting a consulting assignment in Kentucky: as I walked into the facility, there appeared my name in lights — truly, in lights! — "Welcome, Dr. Susan Murphy." I couldn't wait to start working with them.

## PHYSICIAN ORIENTATION TOPICS

A good orientation program for physicians can increase retention, morale, productivity, and loyalty, and can optimize coding and documentation. In a traditional model of physician orientation, the established physician introduces the eager, young physician to his or her nurse, points out the new physician's three exam rooms, and lets them know about the established physician's upcoming two-week vacation in Europe. The hope is that when the established physician returns, the new physician will know how to find the closest emergency room, be familiar with the local specialists, and understand the peculiarities of the office staff. All this accomplished without a lot of pesky questions for the senior doc, right? Well, the problem with this orientation model is that it doesn't work. Instead, it takes much longer for a new physician to become oriented to the practice and takes longer for him/her to feel like an integral part of the practice.[1]

Dr. Grimshaw from the Austin Regional Clinic has developed a physician orientation program that is available for download one time for personal, noncommercial reference through the American Academy of Family Physicians at www.aafp.org/fpm/20010400/39tail.html. Dr. Grimshaw initially developed the program for the Austin Regional Clinic, which has 125 providers, 50 of whom are family practice physicians. According to Dr. Grimshaw, this program could easily be adopted by a practice of any size with any specialty focus.

The program establishes structure around some strategic goals for new physicians:

> A visit-frequency target for new physicians is set: 25 visits per day (twenty-one 15-minute visits and four 30-minute physicals) within the first 7 to 8 weeks;

> New physicians are expected to have between 30 percent and 70 percent same-day appointment availability;

> Physicians' coding and documentation are reviewed after one and four months of employment as part of the program; and

> New physicians receive guidance through a mentoring program and short vignettes about various practice management issues.

The physicians developed single-page, practice management pearls to advise new physicians and increase consistency in the clinic. They chose the topics of pearls based on which subjects prompted the most questions, problems, or complaints from new physicians in the past. The pearls include:

> Angry patients;
> Charting;
> Coding;
> Discharging patients from the clinic;
> Manipulative patients;
> Patients with lists;
> Phone-message management;
> Physicals;

➤ Physician-patient communication;

➤ Poor outcomes and unexpected deaths;

➤ Procedures;

➤ Referring patients to the after-hours clinic;

➤ Refills;

➤ Same-day appointments;

➤ Specialty phone advice;

➤ Utilization management; and

➤ Workers' compensation.

The clinic also identifies and recruits specific mentors for physicians prior to their arrival who are asked to be available by phone and to meet occasionally with new physicians in nonclinical settings, such as a lunch or dinner off-site. In addition to the formal system, the department chief, clinic manager, and administrative representatives make scheduled contact with the new doctors through phone calls or drop-by visits at lunch to provide reinforcement and positive feedback.[1]

## POSITIVE RESULTS

The Austin Regional Clinic has experienced positive results because of this orientation/integration program. Productivity is up "dramatically," documentation is complete, and undercoding of services has been uncovered. In addition, the practice management pearls are being shared with other specialties, and morale has significantly improved.

## SUMMARY

In order to attract, retain, and integrate new team members into your organization, it's important that they believe they are welcomed and that they can be productive and successful. By providing a carefully planned orientation process, you can create a culture where team members and patients can thrive.

## CHAPTER PRESCRIPTIONS

➤ Many team members believe that an orientation is overwhelming and boring. Create a positive and inclusive orientation process for your new hires.

➤ Make team members aware of the overall organization and their place within it. It's imperative that new hires feel as if they "fit" into the structure and that their presence within the organization is pivotal.

➤ Don't allow new team members to feel lost and unwanted. Provide a thorough and meaningful orientation. Ask the senior management team what they want the new recruits to know about their jobs and the organization. Remember that you're building an organization — each member needs to work with the others to achieve success.

➤ Provide effective orientation so the new recruit will feel valued and will be aware of the new position's responsibilities. When provided with such a positive environment, the team member will want to thrive and succeed.

## REFERENCES

[1] R. Grimshaw, "Tailoring New Physicians to Fit Your Practice," *Family Practice Management* 8 (April 2001): 39–43.

## CHAPTER 5

# Developing Team Member Performance Plans

A colleague of mine, a psychologist, has spent 20 years working at one of the most prestigious medical centers in the country. When I called Marilyn to interview her for this chapter, she told me that she has never received feedback on her performance. Each year she gets surprised by a COLA (cost of living adjustment) to her paycheck. She supposes that she's doing an OK job because no one has given her negative feedback. "It's the old 'no news is good news' scenario," she sighed.

This is not an isolated situation. From my experience, there are many medical groups, large and small, that don't have a formal performance management process. Many have job descriptions, and those descriptions include the phrase "other duties as assigned."

In many other medical groups, some of the components for performance management are present but not connected. For example, most staff have job descriptions and their managers conduct performance appraisals year after year. Staff then create performance plans, and often go to training so they can develop skills. Everyone works long, hard hours. There are activities like planning, budgeting, perhaps even board of directors retreats. However, all too often, these activities are done in a vacuum — without being tied directly to the mission, values, and goals of the organization.

Let's look at an example that contrasts two types of managers; one type focuses the team members on activities, and the other focuses on accomplishments and goals.

## THE BEEKEEPERS AND THEIR BEES[1]

Once upon a time, there were two beekeepers who each had a beehive. The beekeepers worked for a company called Bees, Inc. The company's customers loved its honey and wanted the business to produce more honey than it had the previous year. As a result, each beekeeper was told to produce more honey at the same quality. With different ideas about how to do this, the beekeepers designed different approaches to improve the performance of their hives.

The first beekeeper established a bee performance management approach that measured how many flowers each bee visited. At considerable cost to the beekeeper, an extensive measurement system was created to count the flowers each bee visited. The beekeeper provided feedback to each bee at midseason on his/her individual performance, but the bees were never told about the hive's goal to produce more honey so that Bees, Inc., could increase honey sales. The beekeeper created special awards for the bees who visited the most flowers.

The second beekeeper also established a bee performance management approach, but this approach communicated to each bee the goal of the hive — to produce more honey. This beekeeper measured two aspects of their performance: the amount of nectar each bee brought back to the hive and the amount of honey the hive produced. The performance of each bee and the hive's overall performance were charted and posted on the hive's bulletin board for all bees to see. The beekeeper created a few awards for the bees that gathered the most nectar, but also established a hive incentive program that rewarded each bee in the hive based on the hive's production of honey — the more honey produced, the more recognition each bee would receive.

At the end of the season, the beekeepers evaluated their approaches. The first beekeeper found that his hive had indeed increased the number of flowers visited, but the amount of honey produced by the hive had dropped. The queen bee reported that because the bees were so busy trying to visit as many flowers as possible, they limited the amount of nectar they would carry so they could fly faster. Also, because the bees believed they were competing against each other for awards (because only the top performers were recognized), they would not share valuable information with each other (like the location of the flower-filled fields they'd spotted on the way back to the hive) that could have helped improve the performance of all the bees. (After all was said and done, one of the high-performing bees told the beekeeper that if he'd been told that the real goal was to make more honey rather than to visit more flowers, he would have done his work completely differently.) As the beekeeper handed out the awards to individual bees, unhappy buzzing was heard in the background.

The second beekeeper, however, had very different results. Because each bee in the hive was focused on the hive's goal of producing more honey, the bees had concentrated their efforts on gathering more nectar to produce more honey than ever before. The bees worked together to determine the highest nectar-yielding flowers and to create quicker processes for depositing the nectar they'd gathered. They also worked together to help increase the amount of nectar gathered by the poor performers. The queen bee of this hive reported that the poor performers either improved their performance or transferred to another hive. Because the hive had reached its goal, the beekeeper awarded each bee his portion of the hive incentive payment. The beekeeper was also surprised to hear a loud, happy buzz and a jubilant flapping of wings as he rewarded the individual high-performing bees with special recognition.

**MORAL: Measuring and recognizing accomplishments rather than activities — and giving back to worker bees — often improve results of the hive.**

## OVERALL GOAL OF PERFORMANCE MANAGEMENT

To me, the second beekeeper in this "Beekeepers and Their Bees" story models performance management at its best. He systematically developed a high-performing team that produced extraordinary results, received rewards for its accomplishments, and enjoyed the ride!

The overall goal of performance management is to ensure that the whole organization and all of its subsystems, including its managers, staff, departments, processes, and systems, are working together in an optimum fashion to achieve the results desired by the organization. It links the work of each manager and team member to the mission of his or her department as well as to the overall mission of the organization. All team members play a key role in the success of your organization. Just as in the "Beekeepers and Their Bees," story, how well you manage the performance of your team members directly affects not only the performance of the individual team member, but also the performance of your entire organization.

## WHAT IS PERFORMANCE MANAGEMENT?

A good performance management system focuses on achieving results by aligning the performance of all team members with the organizational goals. Performance management is a systematic approach for managing employees and involves planning, monitoring, developing, appraising, rewarding, and improving performance in support of the organizational mission, values, and goals.

Performance management works to achieve consensus, cultivate continuous improvement, support relationships, and ensure that the entire organization is focused on achieving the desired results. It encourages the team to focus on results and accomplishments, not just activities and busyness.

It's a dynamic process that cascades throughout the organization, in every department and in every individual. The ultimate goal of a performance management system is improved organizational performance. An effective performance management system achieves several outcomes, including motivation and retention of talent as well as improved profit, performance, quality, customer service, morale, and efficiency.

Performance management is the systematic continuing process of:

1. Planning work and setting expectations;
2. Continually monitoring performance;
3. Developing the capacity to perform;
4. Periodically rating performance in a summary fashion; and
5. Rewarding good performance.

## PERFORMANCE BENEFITS FOR MANAGERS, TEAM MEMBERS, AND ORGANIZATIONS

Performance management provides the structure for managers to serve as mentors and coaches, and allows them to offer support, encouragement, and guidance in a systematic way. For staff, it provides a framework in which to operate. Most team members welcome some structure as long as it isn't too constraining. When team members are clear about what's expected of them and have the necessary support to contribute efficiently and productively, their sense of purpose, self-worth, and motivation will increase.

## FIVE KEY COMPONENTS OF PERFORMANCE MANAGEMENT

Many managers have been practicing effective performance management naturally during all their supervisory lives, even without formal training in this important area. Others have only been doing one component of this process — that of periodically assigning ratings to the team members's performance. Compared to the other four components, rating performance is the least important part.

Let's look at these five key components more carefully (these are illustrated in Exhibit 5.1).

### Planning

In effective organizations, work is planned in advance. The planning process means setting performance expectations and goals for the organization, the departments, and the individuals. These goals cascade throughout the organization, and each is congruent with the vision, mission, and values of the organization. High-performing organizations get staff at all levels involved in the planning process to ensure that they understand the goals of the entire organization, how their roles and responsibilities fit in with all the organizational goals, what needs to be done, why it needs to be done, and how well it should be done. Performance standards should be SMART — specific, measurable, achievable, results-oriented, and time-bound.

### Monitoring

How well the team members are performing their roles and responsibilities and handling assignments and projects are monitored continually in effective organizations. Effective managers are consistently measuring performance and providing ongoing feedback to team members on their progress toward reaching their goals. By monitoring continually, managers can identify performance that is not goal-oriented and provide assistance so that the team member can get back on track before bad habits are formed. Habits become engrained

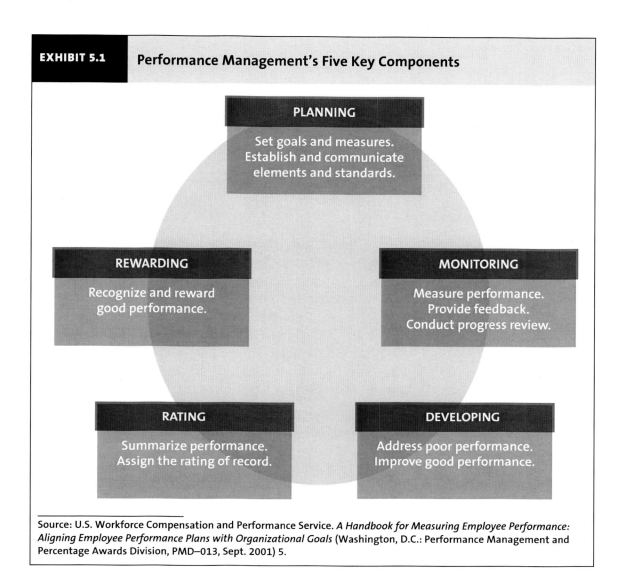

**EXHIBIT 5.1** **Performance Management's Five Key Components**

PLANNING
Set goals and measures. Establish and communicate elements and standards.

REWARDING
Recognize and reward good performance.

MONITORING
Measure performance. Provide feedback. Conduct progress review.

RATING
Summarize performance. Assign the rating of record.

DEVELOPING
Address poor performance. Improve good performance.

Source: U.S. Workforce Compensation and Performance Service. *A Handbook for Measuring Employee Performance: Aligning Employee Performance Plans with Organizational Goals* (Washington, D.C.: Performance Management and Percentage Awards Division, PMD–013, Sept. 2001) 5.

after 21 days, so it's important for managers to provide monitoring and FAST (frequent, accurate, specific, timely) feedback to their team members.

## Developing

In effective organizations, managers identify individuals' developmental needs. Team members receive additional training to learn new skills and handle assignments with higher levels of responsibility. Providing team members with training and developmental opportunities encourages good performance, strengthens job-related skills and competencies, and helps team members keep up with new technology and other changes in the workplace. The developing component enables team members to address poor performance and improve good performance. Team members who are Generation Xers and Millennials will stay more engaged when their managers take an interest in their professional development.

### Rating

Summarizing a team member's performance helps with comparing performance over time or across a group of individuals. It is important that organizations know who their best performers are. Rating is based on work performed during an entire appraisal period, and often has a bearing for pay increases, bonuses, and promotions. With ongoing monitoring and feedback, a performance rating should never be a surprise.

### Rewarding

In effective organizations, rewards are often used and are both formal and informal. Rewarding means recognizing individuals for their performance and acknowledging their contributions to the organization's mission and goals. For good managers, recognition is an ongoing, natural part of every day. Rewards can range from a sincere "thank you," a note of appreciation, time off, or a bonus. A study in *Incentive Magazine* found that 57 percent of respondents said they preferred to be recognized by an immediate supervisor, compared to only 21 percent who placed higher value on a presentation from the company president.[2]

## SIGNIFICANT CONNECTION BETWEEN PERFORMANCE MANAGEMENT AND TEAM MEMBER ENGAGEMENT

In chapter 6 "Creating a Coaching Culture" in *Leading, Coaching, and Mentoring the Team* (Book 2 in the Maximizing Performance Management Series), I report the results of a study by researchers Marcus Buckingham and Curt Coffman of the Gallup organization. For their best-selling book, *First, Break All the Rules*,[3] they interviewed 80,000 managers in 400 organizations and found a significant connection between performance management and employee engagement. They established 12 questions that measure the core elements needed to attract, focus, and keep the most talented employees ... and 7 of these elements relate directly to performance management principles!

In another study of 100,000 employees from 2,500 organizations, the Gallup organization pinpointed employee attitudes that are present in highly productive work groups and that relate directly to the rate of employee turnover, customer satisfaction, and productivity. Many of these attitudes reflect effective performance management practices.

Individuals in these highly productive teams report high levels of agreement with the following statements. Notice how these statements relate directly to good performance management:

- I know what is expected of me at work. (planning)
- At work, I have the opportunity to do what I do best every day. (planning)

➤ In the last six months, someone at work has talked to me about my progress. (monitoring)

➤ There is someone at work who encourages my development. (developing)

➤ I have the materials and equipment I need to do my work right. (developing)

➤ This last year, I have had opportunities at work to learn and grow. (developing)

➤ In the last seven days, I have received recognition or praise for doing good work. (rewarding)

Exhibit 5.2 presents a job description and performance plan for Medical Assistants/Nursing Support in a medical practice. The Camden Group provided this document.

| EXHIBIT 5.2 | Sample Job Description and Performance Plan |
|---|---|

**MEDICAL ASSISTANT/NURSING SUPPORT**
**POSITION DESCRIPTION AND PERFORMANCE PLAN**

**Reports To:** Back Office Supervisor

**Position Summary**

Assist the physicians with the examination and treatment of patients and perform routine tasks needed to keep the clinical office running smoothly.

**Job Responsibilities**

➤ Greets patients and escorts them to the examination and/or procedure rooms. Takes vital signs (pulse, blood pressure, temperature) as well as weight and height; accurately transcribes results in patient's chart.

➤ Assists in completion of forms required by physician prior to examination (e.g., health questionnaires, medical history, etc.).

➤ Removes casts, dressings, and staples as required; prepares patient for examination, test(s), or procedure(s).

➤ Provides instructions when appropriate; obtains signed consent forms when required.

➤ Sets up procedure tray(s).

➤ Notifies physician when patient is ready for examination.

➤ Assists physician with examinations and procedures as needed. Prepares and administers medication as prescribed by the physician.

➤ Labels and color codes blood samples, including packaging of specimens for shipment to appropriate outside labs.

*(continued)*

| EXHIBIT 5.2 (continued) | Sample Job Description and Performance Plan |
|---|---|

➤ Maintains and restocks clinical supplies for back office (e.g., examination and procedure rooms) in addition to inventory control and generating monthly inventory list.

➤ Organizes and keeps a running inventory of medications in med rooms and refrigerator (routinely disposing of expired medications as warranted).

➤ Cleans and scrubs down rooms and countertops per clinical policy.

➤ Cleans, packages, and sterilizes instruments and procedure supplies (forceps, etc.).

➤ Tracks all lab results (e.g., calling for cultures, blood type, and lab information) and documents and initials results in chart when hard copy is not available.

➤ Adheres to OSHA [Occupational Safety and Health Administration] guidelines.

➤ Retrieves prescription calls off voice mail at least three times a day and responds within given timeframes.

➤ Reviews charts for next-day appointments; checks for pending lab or diagnostic test results at the end of each business day; obtains said results prior to the patient's scheduled arrival.

➤ Initials and files all patient-related correspondence within 24 hours of receipt.

➤ Ensures all charts are appropriately filed at the end of each business day.

➤ Maintains daily lab and procedure logs; supplies patient insurance information to lab within 24 hours of test.

➤ Records services rendered on fee tickets (lab, etc.) and checks for accuracy.

➤ Highlights physician notes for ancillary tests, surgeries, or specialist referrals ordered and scheduled as directed.

➤ Directs patient to checkout counter.

➤ Performs any other services deemed reasonable by physician or supervisor.

## QUALIFICATIONS

**Experience and Education.** High school diploma or equivalent or completion of certificated medical assistant program preferred. A multitasked professional with at least three years of experience in performing back-office activities in a medical environment.

**Knowledge.** Basic medical back-office procedures and medical terminology; first aid measures; equipment, supplies, and instruments used in a medical office; simple routine clinical laboratory methods; universal blood and body fluid precautions; OSHA rules and regulations; established protocol for storing poisons, narcotics, acids, caustics, and flammable items; restrictions imposed by various managed care carriers; various forms inherent to profession; patient confidentiality regulations.

**Abilities.** Establish and maintain cooperative relationships with staff members and create a responsive, caring environment for patients; respond promptly to physician's direction(s); maintain medical records in a concise and accurate manner; employ correct aseptic techniques in preparation of instruments and equipment; react quickly in emergency situations and maintain current CPR [cardio pulmonary resuscitation] card; recognize and prevent possible safety hazards; ensure proper maintenance of equipment; communicate clearly and facilitate patient education when warranted; act as advocate and assist physician in meeting the physical and mental needs of patient; exercise independent judgment; perform functions that consistently fall within the legal boundaries of profession.

---

*Note:  This description indicates in general terms the type and level of work performed and responsibilities held by the employee(s). Duties described are not to be interpreted as being all-inclusive.*

I acknowledge receipt of this job description and can fulfill all of the requirements of this position.

Signature:_____Date: _____

| Job Description/Summary | Performance Standards[1] | Performance Tracking[2] |
|---|---|---|
| Assist the physicians with the examination and treatment of patients and perform routine tasks needed to keep the clinical office running smoothly. | 10–15 minutes average waiting time in exam room | Patient log and feedback |
| | 5 minutes average exam room turnaround for the next patient | Patient time log |
| | 100% accuracy in clinical forms documentation | Chart audit |
| | 100% compliance in inventory control and standardization | Inventory control log |
| | 100% compliance to clinical operational protocols | Physician and peer feedback |
| | 100% physician satisfaction | Physician feedback |

Note:  Definition

[1] Performance Standards — are expected measures of individual performance

[2] Performance Tracking — are process activities to track achievement of performance standards

## Medical Assistant/Nursing Support: Guidelines for Performance Plan

In Exhibit 5.2, the position description is shown on the first two pages and the performance plan is on the third page. The very beginning of the document shows the position summary that ties the medical assistant to the big picture.

The position summary clearly states that this team member assists the physicians with the examination and treatment of patients and performs routine tasks needed to keep the clinical office running smoothly.

The performance plan has three components:

1. Job description/summary
2. Performance standards
3. Performance tracking

Team members sign this document and acknowledge receipt of the job description and that they can fulfill all of the requirements of the position.

### Checklist for Effective Performance Plan

When developing performance plans, check against these guidelines:[4]

- Are the critical elements truly critical?
- Is the range of acceptable performance clear? Are the performance expectations quantifiable, observable, and/or verifiable?
- Are the standards attainable? Are the expectations reasonable?
- Are the standards challenging?
- Are the standards fair? Are they comparable to expectations for other staff in similar positions?
- Are the standards applicable? Can the appraiser use the standards to appraise performance? Are they measurable?
- Will team members understand what is required?

## OUTCOMES OF THE PERFORMANCE MANAGEMENT SYSTEM

The overall outcomes of the performance management system will cascade throughout the organization as each unit and individual plays its part and accomplishes his or her own goals. The effect on the entire practice structure and operation may include the following major outcomes for the practice:

- **Performance management stabilization** — creating alignment, organizational initiatives and strategy, department goals, individual performance plans;

> ➤ **Organizational performance** — productivity, adaptability, quality;
> ➤ **Team member satisfaction** — motivation, engagement, retention, and loyalty;
> ➤ **Reward systems** — merit pay, variable pay (short- and long-term incentives, including effect on equity-based rewards), recognition; and/or
> ➤ **Development** — succession planning, training, career progression.

Performance and development planning should be conducted:

> ➤ Annually, at the start of each performance cycle;
> ➤ When a new team member is hired and needs clear goals;
> ➤ When a team member is transferred into a new department; and
> ➤ When organization or department plans are completed.

## INTERNAL AND EXTERNAL INFLUENCES

Performance management does not operate in a vacuum. It's a dynamic system that is affected continually by frequent internal and external pressures that throw it off balance. In chapter 1 when I described the Weisbord 6 Box model, after examining the six boxes inside the system and how they influence one another, I explained the impact of the external influences on the system. Each system is influenced by changes in the other systems.

Internal influences can include budget shortfalls, revamping of the organizational structure, changes in business strategy, and staff and management turnover.

External influences can include changes in customer demands, legal challenges, government regulatory changes, labor market shortages, industry characteristics, resource availability, technology, competition, economics, and politics.

## THE DASHBOARD OF ORGANIZATIONAL GOALS: "IF YOU CAN'T MEASURE IT, YOU CAN'T MANAGE IT"

Although dashboards were discussed in chapter 2 "Developing the Organization's Purpose" in *Aligning the Team with Practice Goals* (Book 1 in the Maximizing Performance Management Series), they play an important part in performance management as well, because in effective organizations, the organizational goals cascade throughout every aspect of the organization. Robert S. Kaplan and David P. Norton developed this concept of creating a set of measures that they refer to as a "balanced scorecard";[5] I like to call it a dashboard. These measures give managers a fast but comprehensive view of

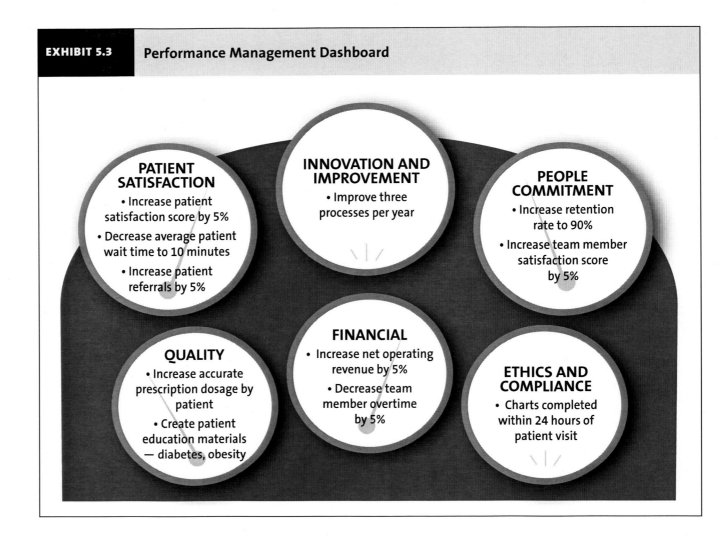

**EXHIBIT 5.3** **Performance Management Dashboard**

**PATIENT SATISFACTION**
• Increase patient satisfaction score by 5%
• Decrease average patient wait time to 10 minutes
• Increase patient referrals by 5%

**INNOVATION AND IMPROVEMENT**
• Improve three processes per year

**PEOPLE COMMITMENT**
• Increase retention rate to 90%
• Increase team member satisfaction score by 5%

**QUALITY**
• Increase accurate prescription dosage by patient
• Create patient education materials — diabetes, obesity

**FINANCIAL**
• Increase net operating revenue by 5%
• Decrease team member overtime by 5%

**ETHICS AND COMPLIANCE**
• Charts completed within 24 hours of patient visit

the organization's performance — like the dashboard in an airplane cockpit, with several dials and indicators. For the complex task of flying an airplane, pilots need detailed information about fuel, air speed, altitude, bearing, and other indicators that summarize the current and predicted environment. Reliance on only one instrument can be fatal.

Leading health care organizations are adopting these dashboards to display their goals and performance measurements. I concur with many experts who believe that if you can't measure it, you can't manage it. Exhibit 5.3 provides an example of a dashboard with short-term SMART performance goals that can be tracked. Exhibit 5.4 is a performance management self-assessment.

## WHY DON'T TEAM MEMBERS PERFORM?

Leadership is the ability to accomplish goals through others, so it's up to the leaders to diagnose what gets in the way. There's not one easy answer about

| EXHIBIT 5.4 | How Good Are You at Performance Management? |
|---|---|

**SELF-ASSESSMENT**

| | | | |
|---|---|---|---|
| 1. Do you understand your organization's mission and goals? | Yes | Somewhat | No |
| 2. Do your department goals support the overall organizational goals? | Yes | Somewhat | No |
| 3. Do you have a written performance plan with clear performance goals for yourself? | Yes | Somewhat | No |
| 4. Do you involve your team members in setting their own written annual performance goals? | Yes | Somewhat | No |
| 5. Do each of your team members clearly understand how they contribute to the overall mission and goals? | Yes | Somewhat | No |
| 6. Do you provide FAST (frequent, accurate, specific, timely) feedback to team members about their performance? | Yes | Somewhat | No |
| 7. Do you meet at least quarterly with each team member to review his/her performance against goals? | Yes | Somewhat | No |
| 8. Do you hold annual performance reviews with each team member, providing a written appraisal and co-creating a performance/career development plan? | Yes | Somewhat | No |

© 2009 Susan A. Murphy, MBA, PhD
NOTE: This exhibit also appears on the CD.

why some individuals don't perform. Below are some of the reasons team members don't perform plus some ideas about what the manager can do to get individuals on track.[6]

➤ **Team members don't know how or what they should do.** The manager can provide training, give clear directions and expectations about the goals, be approachable and encourage questions, and plan projects and assignments together.

➤ **They do not want to do the job.** The manager can talk about the importance of reaching the goals, work with the team member to make the job more stimulating (if possible), and problem-solve together. Do not allow poor performance to continue unchecked.

➤ **There is no negative consequence for poor performance.** The manager can give consistent, honest feedback and appropriate raises. Set consequences, and if improvement doesn't occur, follow through and begin the disciplinary process.

> **The reward or consequence is for not doing what should be done.** The manager can (1) give positive feedback when goals are reached, especially on tough assignments; (2) let team members correct their own errors so they stay goal-focused; and (3) talk about the goals often.

> **Team members think they are doing just fine.** The manager can provide FAST (frequent, accurate, specific, timely) feedback and include self-evaluation by the individual to ensure that he/she is goal focused.

> **Team members think their way, not your way, is better, and it is not.** The manager can explain the benefits of doing things his/her way and include staff in the planning because they are more likely to support changes if they're personally involved in the process.

> **There are obstacles limiting their performance.** The manager can work to remove obstacles by adding resources, training, guidance, or, if appropriate, by seeking cooperation from other managers.

> **Team members fear a negative consequence.** The manager can practice self-control emotionally — no sarcasm or outbursts when errors are made, support individuals as they learn how to correct mistakes, and create an atmosphere of trust and encouragement.

> **Team members think something else is more important.** The manager can prioritize goals with team members and plan with them how to manage important projects.

## CHAPTER PRESCRIPTIONS

> Make your expectations clear to your team members and provide them with the necessary support to execute the goals, whether as individuals, departments, or the organization.

> Make team members a major part of the planning process, and ensure that they understand just how important their goals as individuals are to the implementation of the organization's overriding goals.

> Provide consistent and meaningful feedback to team members so they know what they're doing well and how they might improve on achieving set goals in other areas.

> Look in the mirror! Don't stop at evaluating team members, but be sure to engage in self-assessment at all levels: individually, departmentally, and organizationally.

## REFERENCES

[1] U.S. Workforce Compensation and Performance Service. *A Handbook for Measuring Employee Performance: Aligning Employee Performance Plans with Organizational Goals* (Washington, D.C.: Performance Management and Percentage Awards Division, PMD–013, Sept. 2001).

[2] M. Rauch, "Cash and Praise a Powerful Combo," *Incentive Magazine* (June 1, 2003).

[3] M. Buckingham and C. Coffman, *First, Break All the Rules: What the World's Greatest Managers Do Differently* (New York: Simon & Schuster, 1999).

[4] U.S. Workforce Compensation and Performance Service. *A Handbook for Measuring Employee Performance: Aligning Employee Performance Plans with Organizational Goals* (Washington, D.C.: Performance Management and Percentage Awards Division, PMD–013, Sept. 2001).

[5] R.S. Kaplan and D.P. Norton, "The Balanced Scorecard—Measures that Drive Performance," *Harvard Business Review* (Jan./Feb. 1992).

[6] Adapted from M. Brounstein, *Handling the Difficult Employee: Solving Performance Problems* (Menlo Park, CA: Crisp Publications, 1993).

## CHAPTER 6

# Conducting Performance Appraisals ......................

**As Chris Argyris, Management Guru** said, "People have the capacity to go either way — toward growth or toward stagnation. The design of the system in which they work can significantly influence which way they go, and how far."

## NO SURPRISES

There should never be any surprises during a performance appraisal. Throughout the year, the effective leader has been giving FAST feedback to each team member. This frequent, accurate, specific, and timely feedback lets the team member know when performance is aligned with goals and when it is not. Chapter 2 "The Role of Leaders" and chapter 3 "Leading Through Change," in *Leading, Coaching, and Mentoring the Team* (Book 2 in the Maximizing Performance Management Series) provide specific examples of how to give goal-focused feedback to team members as well as information about the "educable moment" — the time immediately following an action when behavior can best be reinforced.

## FEEDBACK ONCE A YEAR IS NOT EFFECTIVE

Giving feedback once a year at a performance appraisal and expecting an individual's behavior to change has the same effect as dieting once a year on your birthday and expecting to lose weight. Effective leaders provide coaching all year long, so the annual performance appraisal is only one part of the entire performance management system. I believe that one of the most important effects of the performance appraisal is that team members are made aware of the significance of the contribution they are expected to make and what those expectations are. When properly and fairly conducted, the performance appraisal process can increase a team member's sense of personal investment in the organization, strengthen the relationship between the leader and team member, protect the organization legally, enhance the culture of the organization, and align the team member's performance with organizational goals. When conducted poorly, the opposite can occur and work against the leader, the team member, and the organization.

## PLANNING AND PREPARATION

Performance planning begins at the initial preemployment interview when goals, expectations, and values are discussed. The annual performance appraisal is a formal continuation of those discussions.

An effective performance appraisal has four attributes:

1. It is a **formal discussion** between a team member and his/her supervisor.

2. It is a detailed examination of how the team member is **currently performing** on the job.

3. It is a means of determining how the team member can perform more effectively in **the future** and ensuring his/her **continued professional growth and development.**

4. It is a **beneficial** process for the team member, the supervisor, and the organization as a whole.

By *formal* discussion, I don't mean to imply that it's a "formality." A performance appraisal requires careful planning and preparation; it cannot be handled effectively in a casual chat. It is a discussion that occurs at prescribed intervals and follows a specified form specific to your organization. It is not a cursory review. The manager and team member look at the team member's current level of performance in achieving goals and at the quality of that performance, and then determine the reasons (positive or negative) for that level. For example, if one individual is performing a task better than all the other team members, determining the reasons for that individual's success may help improve the others' performance.

It's important to remember that appraisals aren't just a review of the past but are also a guide to the future. To be effective, performance appraisals must chart a path to the future with plans to increase performance in some areas, if appropriate, as well as begin a process that assists managers in identifying talent, rewarding achievement, and encouraging professional growth. Many organizations now say, "Our employees are our most important asset." I like Michael Eisner's quote when he was the chief executive officer of the Walt Disney Company, "Our inventory goes home every night." The key to achieving the benefits of a successful performance appraisal system is the linking of the team member's skills and achievements to the goals of his/her department, and ultimately to the achievement of the organization's goals and mission.

## MANAGERS INITIATE PROCESS

Managers have the responsibility to initiate the performance review process and to schedule the upcoming meeting. I continue to be disappointed with many managers who are late in initiating this process. Team members usually know, to the day, when their year is up and their appraisals and raises are due. Although staff often fear the process, they want feedback from their manager and then to receive their increase. Some team members complain to me that their managers are always late. Even though the salary increase is often retroactive to their anniversary date, the team members don't want to be the ones to initiate the conversation about the late performance review because they're concerned the manager may score them lower because they're behaving like a pest. Resentment builds and the review meeting becomes even more tense.

## TEAM MEMBER UPDATES JOB DESCRIPTION AND SELF-ASSESSMENT

Invite the team member to suggest any updates to the job description roles and responsibilities and to complete a self-assessment prior to the meeting. I have always encouraged the team member to return the self-assessment to the manager before the meeting, which allows the manager to see how the person views his/her own performance. As a manager, you can gain valuable insight into what an individual is thinking and use this to craft the discussion at the performance review meeting.

## MANAGERIAL PREPARATION

I recommend that you complete the evaluation form at one sitting, and then review it at a later time. Edit and then reedit. Every word is important to the team member, and I guarantee that many of your team members will read their reviews several times — especially any portion you rate less than "excellent." Review the team member's job description, performance goals, and rules of conduct, and assess his/her job performance against these criteria. Review the team member's history, including job skills, training, experience, and special or unique qualifications. Note any variances in the individual's performance that need to be discussed, and ensure that you provide specific examples for every area. The next step is to review what you have written and check for any biases or inflammatory wording. Then determine rating and merit increase.

As you are reviewing the team member's performance before the meeting, I recommend you consider questions from Rummler and Brache.[1] If any of the six statements can be answered "no," you may need to include that discussion in the performance review meeting. There could be some system problems that are impeding the team member's ability to excel in his or her position.

1. Do the performers understand the job goals (standards they are expected to meet)?

2. Do the performers have sufficient resources, clear signals and priorities, and a logical job design?

3. Are the performers rewarded for achieving the job goals?

4. Do the performers know if they are meeting the job goals?

5. Do the performers have the necessary knowledge/skill to achieve the job goals?

6. If the performers were in an environment in which the five questions were answered "yes," do they have the physical and mental capacity to achieve the goals?

## PITFALLS TO AVOID

It's easy to succumb to pitfalls that may skew an honest assessment of the team member's job performance. For example, you may give too much weight to recent events that have occurred that don't represent the team members's behavior during the entire year. Additionally, there are some team members whom managers like better — people who have similar values, interests, and personality traits. It's important to evaluate job performance and not play favorites. Another pitfall is called the "halo" or "horns" effect that occurs when the manager is influenced by a recent single event involving the individual. The manager may also be tempted to be lenient and rate everyone higher than deserved in order to make it easier to get through the process — as well as make it easier for the team to like the manager. It's also tempting to rate all the team members similarly and place everyone in the middle of the scale.

Other examples of pitfalls can be a bias or prejudice that the manager holds against the team member that has nothing to do with job performance. These prejudices could include religion, education, family background, age, or gender. Sometimes a team member may have excelled or performed poorly in one or two areas, and this may trigger the manager to give an unbalanced evaluation based on those few areas. Another pitfall to an effective performance review process is when the team member is not allowed enough time to complete the self-assessment.

# THE APPRAISAL INTERVIEW

The appraisal interview is one of the manager's most important meetings with the team member for the entire year. Team members often dread this meeting and need the manager to make the meeting private and as comfortable as possible. Schedule one to one-and-a-half hours of uninterrupted time for the meeting. Following is an outline of how to best conduct the meeting so you and the individual both have the opportunity to discuss and review all that you both need and wish to.

1. **Greet the team member and establish rapport immediately.** The individual is probably apprehensive and will welcome your gesture to establish a warm climate. It's important to keep in mind that your opening remarks set the tone for the rest of the meeting.

2. **Explain the purpose and benefits of the performance review process.** Ask if the person has any questions or comments before you start.

3. **Request the team member give his/her opinion of performance since the last appraisal.** Ask where the person believes s/he's doing well and areas where s/he might improve. Seeking a team member's opinion of his/her performance shows that you, as the manager, respect his/her contribution, expertise, and knowledge. This can give you an accurate picture of how the team member is doing and may uncover some problem areas where you can help.

   Ask open-ended questions to gain information — who, what, when, where, how, why, describe, tell me. Don't talk too much during the assessment — this is the individual's time to present his/her evaluation of performance.

4. **Present your own evaluation of the team member's performance and give recognition for accomplishments since the last review.** Avoid terms such as *always* and *never*. A key to raising performance levels is motivation, and one key to motivation is recognition. By providing specific examples of performance where you believe that your team member deserves recognition, the individual will feel appreciated because s/he knows you've "caught them doing something right," as Ken Blanchard preaches.[2]

   Confirm where you agree with your team member during the performance review. Where you disagree, give your own views with specific examples. Let the team member see that you are interested in helping him/her succeed.

5. **Seek your team member's input on one or two performance areas that s/he believes could be developed.** Compare the individual's responses with your choices, then negotiate together to

develop an action plan. Check his/her understanding and reaction. Psychologists indicate that when an individual is faced with more than two areas in which performance should be improved, that person becomes defensive and feels the supervisor is being critical instead of supportive. This can endanger the performance review and lead to a nonmotivational discussion.

6. **Ask your team member if there is anything that you could be doing to help him/her in being more effective at work.** This can provide the manager with some feedback of how to be more effective with the team.

7. **Review with your team member the benefits of the performance review and summarize key points to ensure understanding by both manager and staff member.** Review the overall performance, stressing the areas where the individual is excelling.

8. **End the performance review with a positive, motivating message.** By ending with upbeat, encouraging words, the team member returns to work in a positive frame of mind.

Knowing that your manager is on your side can be a powerful motivator. By conducting an honest, respectful performance appraisal that is focused on the goals of the department and the organization, you are aligning your team member's performance with the organizational goals. Exhibit 6.1 provides a performance appraisal checklist for managers.

## HOW TO PROVIDE FEEDBACK DURING APPRAISAL

Some general guidelines for giving feedback include:

- Focus on relevant performance and behavior, not the person;
- Focus on specific, observable behavior, not on general impressions;
- Avoid loaded terms that produce an emotional reaction or cause defensiveness;
- Focus on areas over which the person can exercise some control or for which s/he can use the feedback to improve;
- When encountering defensive reactions, deal with reactions rather than try to convince, reason, or supply other information; and
- End on a positive note. Focus on keeping the self-esteem of both parties intact.

## 360-DEGREE FEEDBACK

The 360-degree feedback method is a tool that provides team members the opportunity to receive feedback from their manager, three to eight peers, direct reports, and customers. The team member also responds to a self-assessment for

| EXHIBIT 6.1 | Performance Appraisal Checklist for Managers |
| --- | --- |

**I. PREPARATION BY MANAGER**

☐ Review job performance against mutually understood expectations with job responsibilities, goals, rules of conduct.

☐ Avoid pitfalls: bias, recent events vs. year-long performance, playing favorites, "halo"/"horn" effect, too lenient, everyone the same, unbalanced review.

☐ Review team member's background: work experience, skills, and training.

☐ Evaluate team member's strengths and development areas for goal setting.

☐ Ensure team member has time to prepare self-assessment.

☐ Schedule time for private, uninterrupted discussion.

**II. CONDUCTING A PERFORMANCE APPRAISAL MEETING**

☐ Conduct the meeting by creating a private, comfortable environment; reviewing purpose of performance review; both to participate in goal setting.

☐ Listen closely as team member conducts self-assessment of job responsibilities, strengths, accomplishments, areas for development. Ask open-ended questions.

☐ Keep focus on job performance. Discuss job responsibilities, team member's strengths, accomplishments, development areas. Give examples for each area.

☐ Agree on development, set SMART goals and where support is needed.

**III. CONCLUDING THE MEETING**

☐ Summarize discussion.

☐ Give team member an opportunity to make additional suggestions.

☐ End on a positive, friendly, harmonious note.

☐ Record commitments and points for follow-up.

**IV. EVALUATING THE MEETING**

☐ What I did well and could have done better.

☐ What I learned about team member and his/her job.

☐ What I learned about myself and my job.

NOTE: This exhibit also appears on the CD.

comparison. This format allows individuals to understand their effectiveness as employees, coworkers, and managers. I've been involved in several 360-degree assessments, and I know firsthand how critical it is that this form of feedback system be established in a careful, methodical manner that includes training and support for all involved. When implemented well, 360-degree feedback enables people in organizations to better serve customers, enhance interpersonal skills, and develop their careers. This kind of feedback can provide each individual important insight about the skills and behaviors valued in the organization to accomplish the mission, vision, and values and to align performance with the organizational goals. I recommend that the 360-degree feedback be separate from the formal performance appraisal system. When first rolled out, this form of feedback works best as a professional development tool. Sure, it can identify areas for improvement; however, I've seen it work best initially when it is not associated directly with compensation changes.

## CAREER DEVELOPMENT QUESTIONS

Research indicates that more than 60 percent of staff, no matter what age, gender, or generation, want career development opportunities. During the performance review, it can be a good time to ask your team members some questions about their career goals. Some questions about career level performance goals include:

> What job/occupation would you like to have in three to five years?

> What skills, experiences, and competencies are required by the job?

> What are you planning to do to prepare yourself for that job?

> How can I support your efforts?

## CHAPTER PRESCRIPTIONS

> Ensure that team members are made aware of the importance of the contribution expected of them and exactly what those expectations are.

> Remember that an effective performance appraisal process can increase a team member's sense of worth and investment within the organization, strengthen the relationship between employer and team member, enhance the culture of the organization, and align team member performance with organizational goals.

> Approach each performance appraisal as a discussion that occurs at assigned and expected intervals and follows a specific set of rules.

> Team member appraisals are useful in assessing the individual's past performance, but should also be used to set clear goals for the future. Therefore, have the team member fill out a self-assessment prior to the meeting so that the manager can address issues that are specific to each team member's needs. It's also helpful to have a sense of how the team member views his/her work performance before the meeting.

➤ Provide meaningful and accurate feedback for your team members — if you just tell them what they want to hear, you may be liked, but your organization is sure to suffer.

➤ People are always more apt to be open to criticism when they are also told what they are doing well. Be sure to hone in on what you feel the team member is bringing to the organization, and then discuss areas for improvement — use the organizational goals as a tool for aligning each team member within the practice.

## REFERENCES

[1] G.A. Rummler and A.P. Brache, *Improving Performance: How to Manage the White Space on the Organizational Chart* (San Francisco: Jossey-Bass, 1995).

[2] K.H. Blanchard and S. Johnson, *The One Minute Manager* (New York: Morrow, 1982).

## CHAPTER 7

# Summary......................................................

Team members are your most valuable asset — when you nurture and grow your team, you nurture and grow your practice. As described in chapter 1, every practice is a dynamic system made up of six subsystems — all of which must be in balance to consistently support the practice goals. If one or more of these subsystems is weak and thus does not support the practice goals, there cannot be maximum performance from the team members.

This third book in the *Maximizing Performance Management Series* is a how-to guide for evaluating two of your organization's subsystems — "Rewards" and "Structure." In *Building and Rewarding Your Team,* you learned that designing a compensation and incentive structure for physicians is not for the faint hearted. You also learned that involving physicians in strategic planning, goal setting, and developing performance expectations is important, and the critical step that follows is translating those values and priorities into a reward system for physicians and staff. You've explored the rewards and recognition needs of an engaged team and how to evaluate your compensation system for effectiveness.

While studying the "Structure" subsystem, you've discovered the five important performance management components needed to align team members with the practice's mission, values, and goals. An effective performance management system serves to motivate, engage, and increase staff retention – as well as achieve practice goals of quality, productivity, patient satisfaction, and morale. You've learned that when there is an open position, your initial steps are to ask questions about the organizational structure, such as whether the position should be filled and, if so, with what skill set. Additionally you've explored the significance of creating an effective performance appraisal system that measures and recognizes accomplishments rather than activities.

*Building and Rewarding Your Team* and the other three books in this comprehensive, results-oriented series provide a road map and prescriptions to take you and your practice to the next level and beyond.

## About the Author

∙ ∙ ∙ ∙ ∙ ∙ ∙ ∙ ∙ ∙ ∙ ∙ ∙ ∙ ∙ ∙ ∙ ∙ ∙ ∙ ∙ ∙ ∙ ∙ ∙ ∙ ∙ ∙ ∙ ∙ ∙ ∙ ∙ ∙ ∙ ∙ ∙ ∙ ∙ ∙ ∙ ∙ ∙ ∙ ∙ ∙ ∙ ∙ ∙ ∙ ∙ ∙ ∙ ∙ ∙ ∙ ∙

Susan A. Murphy, MBA, PhD, is President of Business Consultants Group, Inc., based in Rancho Mirage, California. Dr. Murphy's extensive professional background combines the worlds of corporate leadership, academia, and management consulting. She has served as an executive in two Fortune 500 Corporations as well as on the graduate faculty at the University of San Francisco. She has also provided international management consulting for 20 years to more than 250 health care organizations and businesses. Clients include Stanford University Department of Pediatrics, Kaiser Permanente, Jet Propulsion Lab (JPL), Tenet Healthcare Corp., the U.S. Air Force, and the Medical Group Management Association.

Passionate about leadership, mentoring, and teaching individuals about gender and generational differences, Dr. Murphy thrives on serving as a catalyst for breakthrough team performance. She has coauthored numerous books including: *In the Company of Women, Conversations on Success, 4genR8tns: Succeeding with Colleagues, Cohorts & Customers,* and *Leading a Multi-Generational Workforce. In the Company of Women,* coauthored with Dr. Pat Heim, has been featured on *Good Morning, America,* the British Broadcasting Corporation, and usatoday.com, as well as in *Time Magazine.* The book was selected as Harvard Business School's "Book of the Month" and has been translated into several languages.

As a keynote speaker, Dr. Murphy is known for her "Wit and Wisdom." Audiences everywhere appreciate her humorous style and useful techniques, as she combines research and theory with real-life experiences. In 2004, Vanderbilt University honored Dr. Murphy with a Lifetime Achievement Award.

# Index

# *About the CD*

. . . . . . . . . . . . . . . . . . . . . . . . . . . . . . . . . . . . . . . . . . . . . . . . . . . . .

Included with this book is a CD-ROM containing tools, helping mechanisms, and case studies.

## HOW TO USE THE FILES ON YOUR CD-ROM

The CD-ROM presents tools and case studies in Microsoft®Word and PDF formats. You can change Microsoft®Word documents, but you can't change PDFs. You must have Microsoft®Word and Adobe® Reader® installed on your hard drive to use the CD-ROM. To adapt any Microsoft®Word file to your own practice, simply follow the instructions below. The CD-ROM will work on Windows and Mac platforms.

### Microsoft®Word Instructions for Windows

1. Insert the CD in your CD-ROM drive.
2. Double-click on the "My Computer" icon, and then double click on the CD drive icon.
3. Double-click on the folder named "Maximizing Performance Management."
4. The folders you see are organized into the same categories as those in the book—Tools/Helping Mechanisms and Case Studies. Double click on the appropriate subfolder, and then double click to open the Microsoft®Word or PDF file you wish to download.
5. If you have trouble reading the Microsoft®Word files, click on "View", and then "Normal."
6. To adapt the Microsoft®Word file, you must save it to your hard drive first, renaming it if you like. After you have resaved it, the file can be edited.